Nurses' Clinical Decision Making

Russell Gurbutt

Senior Lecturer Health Informatics
Lancashire School of Health and Post Graduate Medicine
University of Central Lancashire

Foreword by

Carl Thompson

Radcliffe Publishing
Oxford • Seattle

Radcliffe Publishing Ltd
18 Marcham Road
Abingdon
Oxon OX14 1AA
United Kingdom

www.radcliffe-oxford.com
Electronic catalogue and worldwide online ordering facility.

British Library Cataloguing in Publication Data

A catalogue record for this book is available from the British Library.

ISBN-10 1 84619 037 1
ISBN-13 978 1 84619 037 7

Typeset by Anne Joshua & Associates, Oxford
Printed and bound by TJ International Ltd, Padstow, Cornwall

Contents

Foreword

The clinical decisions of nurses and the quality of the judgements that inform them are at the heart of modern health services. Since Florence Nightingale, nurses have engaged in the selection of choices for and with patients. Often this contribution has been downplayed or classed as 'unofficial' or 'informal'. This situation is changing. Nurses have begun to take on decision-making roles and to embrace the opportunities for improved patient care that these roles offer. Moreover, the delivery and organisation of services themselves have begun to be shaped by the recognition that, at least for some patients, nurses provide as good, and in some cases better, care than their medical colleagues. Areas such as tissue viability, diabetes care, stroke rehabilitation and heart failure management have all seen significant benefits accrue when nurses are freed up to lead, exercise their judgement and make decisions. In the UK, the vision of the modern nurse as someone who can bridge outmoded and outdated distinctions between 'caring' and 'curing' is fast becoming a reality. Initiatives such as nurse prescribing, the ordering (and just as importantly, the interpretation) of diagnostic tests and spread of nurse-led 'first contact' care all mean that seamless provision of services is at least on the policy agenda.

Of course, with these roles and opportunities for professional development come great responsibilities. Approximately one in ten patients coming into contact with acute healthcare endure some form of adverse event, of which around half are due to errors and have an avoidable component to them. Nurses, as a central part of the healthcare team, are implicated in these statistics. Areas such as responding to deteriorating physical observations (60% of cardiac arrests have documented abnormal observations), diagnosing risks and communicating those risks to patients and medical colleagues, as well as assessing the preferences of patients for the choices they face are all areas in which nursing can improve (and thankfully is improving).

Russell Gurbutt's contribution to this improvement is to explore, describe and highlight the hidden and the discrete in nurses' decision making. This is an important contribution, for if we are to start really improving the choices that healthcare professionals make then the first step on this journey is to know something about the reality of the types of decisions and judgements that are involved, the contexts in which they are made, the points of departure from the rational or what we know about how people *should* make decisions, and the ways in which groups of decision makers interact. Only when we have this information is it possible to adapt normative models of decision making to clinical practice. An analogy to wine making is possible here: producing great wine depends in part on knowledge of the terroir (or terrain, micro culture, local climates and soil composition) in an area. What Russell has produced in this text is a map of nursing's decision making 'terroir'. Like any journey in which progress is mapped there are some uncomfortable moments: the negative impact of workload and limited time on choices; the doctor-nurse 'game' (still so prevalent after being first revealed in the 1960s); and the often woeful inadequacies and inefficiencies of information systems (including nurses' own records) all stand out. However, what this text manages to reveal is that despite this discomfort, there is a richness and depth to the ways in which nurses describe, and are seen to enact, their decisions and judgements.

This book provides a fine start point for all those interested in enhancing the decision making capacity of nurses and improving their contribution to patient care. I have no hesitation in commending this book to all those who want to improve their knowledge of the realities of decision making from a nurse's perspective.

Dr Carl Thompson D. Phil (Social Policy) BA (Hons) RN
Senior Lecturer Health Sciences
University of York
Editor *Evidence Based Nursing*
July 2006

Preface

Clinical work is complex and takes place in a complex environment that centres around individuals who themselves are physically, socially and spiritually complex. Clinical work also involves multiple participants (nurses, doctors, patients, physiotherapists, occupational therapists and pharmacists, to name just a few) who in the course of a day's work can make scores of decisions. Some of these are deliberatively thought out whilst others are seemingly made at a subconscious level, often described as intuitive decisions. How then can we make sense of the complex real world of clinical practice to the extent that we can recognise how decisions are made and know whether or not these decisions satisfy a range of evaluation measures?

This book offers a way of finding answers to these questions. Its origins lie in having to examine complaints made about practitioners' decisions in the real world of clinical practice. In it I draw upon and use the findings of a research study of nurses' clinical decision making as a framework to guide your examination of how you, the reader, make decisions, evaluate decisions, learn about decision making, and understand notions of developing experience and expertise in decision making. I do not claim that this is a universal account of how all nurses make decisions, but I do offer this particular account as a means of drawing attention to the centrality of nurses' clinical decision making in their work.

Decision making is not fully understood, and there is still much to study about how different groups of practitioners make decisions, and about multi-disciplinary decision making and the interplay between the participants and the organisational setting in decision making. Having acknowledged this, we still need to take a proactive approach to understanding clinical decision making in the complex real world of healthcare service delivery. This book is a step on the trajectory of a work in progress that takes up the baton of decision enquiry that has been reported to date, and will no doubt be handed on to a new generation of enquiring practitioners.

My decision to write the book is grounded in experience of clinical decision making and research into nurses' decision making alongside the education of nurses, doctors, social workers and therapists. This has specifically included teaching decision making, health informatics and risk management modules as well as being course leader for adult nurse training. The latter role highlighted the need to recognise decision making as part of the nurse's role and to seek ways to prepare trainees to be competent decision makers and then continue to develop their expertise after registration. I hope, therefore, that you enjoy reading the book and that it provokes you to examine how decisions are made in your workplace, their context, the participants and your role in this process. Above all I hope that it stimulates reflection on how you know patients and act in response to such knowledge.

Russell Gurbutt
July 2006

About the author

Russell Gurbutt has been a registered nurse for almost 20 years and has clinical experience in the public and private sectors, including management of a number of NHS hospital ward teams in surgery and medicine. He currently works at the University of Central Lancashire as part of the health informatics team in the School of Health and Postgraduate Medicine. His research interests are in management and clinical decision making.

Acknowledgements

I wish to thank Steve Willcocks, Martin Johnson and Alan Gillies for advice received while undertaking the decision-making study that is referred to in this book. I am also grateful to Gillian Nineham for advice and encouragement to publish the book. Last but not least, thanks to Dawne, Jessica and Thomas Gurbutt, who have lived with this study and the subsequent drafting of the manuscript.

A guide to using this book

This book has been written with particular audiences in mind. These are practitioners who make decisions, those learning to make clinical decisions as part of gaining professional registration, those who monitor decisions, and those involved in pre- and post-registration education of decision makers. The chapters build up a description of how patients are known and how this knowledge is used by nurses to make decisions. A range of questions might be raised as you read through the book and consider the complexity of nurses' clinical decision making. I have included some questions at the end of each chapter in the 'Stop and think' section to facilitate the making of links with your own practice.

Each chapter has the following format:

- introduction
- main text of chapter
- chapter summary box
- 'Stop and think' section.

Chapter 1 Setting the scene: the clinical landscape of decision making

In this chapter I set the scene with regard to clinical decision making and examine developments in the role of nurses as decision makers, and the process, outcomes and context of decision making.

Chapter 2 Making clinical decisions: a model of nurses' decision making

In this chapter I introduce a model of decision making that is used as a framework to guide examination of a range of different features of the process. This model represents how nurses seek and interpret information to generate a narrative about a patient. This is used to identify their needs and choose interventions. The transition from an individual- to a group-owned narrative and way of shaping consensus on how a patient is known is examined.

Chapter 3 The narratives that nurses generate: ways of knowing the patient

In this chapter I focus on how patients can be known in different ways and I explore the implications that this has for the decisions that nurses make.

Chapter 4 Demonstrating narratives: differences between verbal and written narratives

In this chapter I examine the invisibility of much of what nurses know about patients by comparing verbal narratives with their written counterparts in nurses' records.

Chapter 5 The games nurses play: making narratives known to doctors

In this chapter I examine the invisibility of nurses' decision making and how they make their narratives known in order to influence doctors' decisions.

Chapter 6 Narratives and expert decision makers: creating and using narratives

In this chapter I examine how different nurses can be described as inexperienced, experienced and expert, according to the extent to which they can create and use narratives.

Chapter 7 Nurses as decision makers: where next?

This summary draws on the preceding chapters to consider the challenges and opportunities that nurses face in placing knowing the patient at the heart of clinical practice.

Chapter 1

Setting the scene: the clinical landscape of decision making

Introduction • Raising questions • Origins and developments • Knowledge and decision making • Rules and decision making • Assistants in medical decision making • Breakout: developing nurse decision making • Nursing models and decision making • Decision-making enquiry about different types of nurse • Decision-making enquiry about different types of decision • Decision-making enquiry about process • Decision-making enquiry and the use of different terminology • Decision making and problem solving • Decision-making outcomes • Decision-making process • Theoretical explanations • Decision-making context • The clinical landscape • Conclusion • Stop and think

Introduction

If nurses are decision makers, how can their role and practice be explained? Can decision making be taught and are there different levels of decision-making skill? If so, how can expert decision makers be recognised? These are just some of the pertinent questions that need to be asked if we are to recognise and understand the centrality of clinical decision making in nursing practice.

This chapter introduces nurses' decision making. At the outset it considers two clinical incidents which highlight a range of questions that real-world practice raises about decision making. Then selected developments in nurses' decision-making practice are introduced to highlight how the role has developed and subsequently moved away from its medically dominated origins. The contribution of nursing models to the construction of professional identity is used to mark a shift in focus towards nursing decisions. Different types of nurse and nursing decision are explored along with the processes that they use and the descriptive terminology employed. Links between decision making and problem solving are discussed along with explanations of decision outcomes. Different theoretical explanations of the whole process are identified before returning to contemporary accounts of the context of nurses' decision making and its influence on the process.

Throughout the chapter the intention is to show that nurses have a decision-making role and that their practice includes a range of elements (e.g. information seeking, processing, knowledge, outcome). Although theoretical accounts draw these elements together, a unifying theory of decision making does not exist. Figure 1.1 shows how key areas of decision making can be drawn together as a reference to consider where decision-making enquiry has been and can be directed. It incorporates the decision maker(s), decision process, decision outcome and decision-making context. Now let us turn our attention to questions about decision making that can be generated through real-world practice.

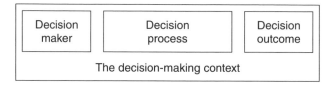

Figure 1.1 A model showing key areas of decision making. The model consists of a decision maker, a decision process, a decision outcome and a decision-making context.

Raising questions

Think about what it is like to go into hospital as a patient, to be drawn into the daily business of a complex service provided by numerous people. These include nurses, therapists, chaplains, doctors, porters, laboratory technicians, chefs, cleaning staff, administrators and managers, to name just a few. As a patient, you have expectations about the service that you think you need, an understanding of the extent of your participation in decision making, and a degree of trust in the decisions that healthcare staff make about your care and treatment. Incidents occur that raise concerns – perhaps a missed medication, overlooked requests or staff seeming to be too busy to stop and chat. A catalogue of small events can lead to a perception that decisions are being made about you but not with you. Some might actually contribute to harm rather than good. Why would this be and how can it be explained? Who is making decisions and, perhaps more importantly, are some decisions being overlooked? Clinical incidents occur in health service delivery. The two scenarios that follow raise interesting questions.[1]

During an evening shift on an understaffed 36-bed stroke rehabilitation ward the nurse in charge was commencing a drug round. She had two care assistants on duty who were busy attending to patients as they worked their way down the ward. The staff nurse glanced down the ward and saw a patient trying to roll over in his bed. She called to him to stop as she anticipated (correctly) that he would fall on to the floor. There was not time to get to his bed, and as he fell out of bed on to the floor, there was an audible crack. His femur had fractured. Three days later he died.

This incident raised many questions. Who had assessed the patient's needs and planned his care? Had a care plan been devised that addressed the need to maintain a safe environment? Should rehabilitating patients be expected to take risks (as people in normal health do) and should it be accepted that falls can happen during the process of regaining independence? Had a decision not been made that ultimately contributed to the patient's death? Sometimes examining practice generates far more questions than answers. Fortunately, not all clinical incidents are as serious as this one. The next story is about a complaint which implied that nurses were omitting to provide adequate care for a patient. At best it was an organisational or resource management problem and at worst an allegation of negligence.

A stroke patient had been convalescing for several weeks on a busy 28-bed rehabilitation ward. The ward was short staffed and the three or four staff on duty on each shift (registered nurses and care assistants) were involved in physically demanding work. The most that they could achieve with each patient during a shift was to attend to their daily needs (such as washing, dressing, feeding and toileting) and help with some physical therapy. A complaint was made by the patient's relative in which it was claimed that the rehabilitation process was too slow. This was attributed to deficits in the nursing care provided. A local enquiry took place to investigate the complaint and provide a written response.

The investigation included discussions with the ward team about their care decisions and examination of their records. Neither of these sources of enquiry provided a satisfactory answer about what was planned and provided, nor did they explain how and why decisions had been made or, as was alleged, over-looked. However, this investigation did generate interest in proposing a study of how registered nurses made clinical decisions. The findings of that study (of nurses in four NHS general medical wards) are used to explain different features of decision making, decision makers and their practice in the chapters of this book. The aftermath of the response to the complaint generated several questions about nurses' decision making. For example, could nurses recognise the range and volume of decisions made in the course of their practice? Could they recognise and explain their decision making? Furthermore, if this could be explained, why did their care records not clearly demonstrate this? Both scenarios require questioning to go beyond asking what happened and who made decisions. The decision-making processes, context, participants and their re-sources are just some of the factors that need to be considered when seeking to find out why and how decisions are made.

Back in the ward a learning opportunity was lost. The pace of work gave little respite to seriously examine practice that at times was on a merry-go-round of trying to match limited resources with ever-increasing demand. There is a saying that 'if we do what we have always done then we will get what we have always got'. How apt – but we need to find a way of stepping aside for a while to examine what it is that nurses do and to learn about their clinical decision making. Why is this? It is so that nurses can know how central decision making is to their role and are able to articulate what it is that they do.

Given that there are often more questions than answers, any simple explan-ations of decision making seem inadequate. Indeed, as was intimated earlier, hospitals are complex organisations involving many people, many interactions, and different processes and information sources. It is not surprising that real-world clinical decision making should be regarded as complex. Some scene setting follows about the development of nurses as decision makers and their decision-making practice.

Origins and developments

There are different claims about the origin of nurse decision-making enquiry. These have included the game theory,[2] which dealt with decision making under uncertain conditions and has been linked to applications in economics and military planning.[3] In contrast, others[4] have favoured an organisational basis in models taken from the field of academic administration to explain management and patient care decisions. These differences reflect a preference for a methodological approach and point of enquiry – for instance, a psychology discipline perspective.[5] The work of Florence Nightingale[6] can be taken as a convenient origin point. In her era the foundations of decision making in contemporary British adult nursing practice were laid. Decision making is implicit within her 1859 text, *Notes on Nursing*, in which she described the nurse's role and linked it to a distinction (made in response to criticism from medical staff) between nursing care and medical cure roles. This had implications with regard to the legitimate scope of nurses' decisions, their knowledge base and decision-making information processing. Although other groups, such as religious orders (especially in Germany), pre-dated Nightingale's response, it was her work that described the role of the nurse in Britain.[7] Nursing care roles were grounded in Nightingale's belief that health was subject to laws of nature which required nurses to *'put the patient in the best condition for nature to act upon him.'* Consequently they had a sick-room management role and observed a patient's health change. In contrast, medical staff were concerned with curative interventions to assist the natural processes of healing. Political legitimacy had been given to medical diagnostic decision making through the 1858 Medical Registration Act, which excluded from medicine the amateur 'physicking' of *'unauthorised practitioners'* who were described as *'wise women, healers, chemists and druggists'*.[8] This rendered diagnostic decision making by nurses illegal, whilst decision-making authority resided with doctors. It was not until the latter part of the twentieth century that economic expediency, policy shifts and professionalisation agendas reshaped the scope of nursing work as far as clinical decision making was concerned.

From Nightingale's day nurses' decisions addressed their duty of being *'in charge of the personal health of another'*,[6] which implied an individual focus (on a patient), acting vicariously (in charge of another's health) and having decision authority (taking charge). As sick-room managers, nurses controlled the physical environment (noise, heat, light, ventilation) and regulated patient activity (mobility, diet, hygiene, toileting) and social issues (access of others and recreation). These translate into contemporary practice as management of the patient in the ward environment, and include clinical governance, risk management and resource management. It is often the nurse who 'owns' the ward, orders equipment, checks stock levels, and ensures that maintenance is periodically undertaken and that sufficient staff are rostered to provide care. All other staff visit the ward, but nurses have a 24-hour presence. Today, as in the 1800s, nurses own the ward and the patients within it. This has not unnaturally led to them wanting to do more than merely observe health change and carry out the instructions of medical staff. They also wanted to diagnose problems, and to do that they needed to develop their knowledge base. Two directions could have been taken. The first was to make medical diagnoses, and the second was to develop a nursing knowledge base and make nursing diagnoses. Both directions have been taken, although at different times, and this has resulted in recent developments in the scope of nurses' work – for example, nurse practitioners and consultant nurses.

Knowledge and decision making

Resistance to nursing development came swiftly when attempts were made to second guess medical diagnoses and threatened medical control.[9] Servitude characterised nursing work, which as far back as 1885 was based on carrying out the doctor's instructions.[10] Whilst upholding a notion of obedience to medical staff, some doctors recognised the value of independent cognitive action, stating that the nurse must demonstrate *'constant obedience and loyalty in fulfilling her prescribed duties, but also . . . much more intelligent co-operation in the treatment of disease'*.[11]

Assumptions about the ability of women to utilise information limited the progress that could be made towards independent decision making. Far from not knowing anything about the laws of health in Nightingale's era, nurses sought to acquire clinical knowledge. This was sufficient for a doctor in 1925 to acknowledge a problem of *'preventing nurses from attempting to acquire knowledge'* and to recommend that doctors use *'our influence to prevent the illegitimate use of such knowledge'*.[9] Nurses' desire for knowledge could not be stemmed, and opinion was divided about what to do, from regulating its use to espousing a thorough understanding of *'scientific detail'*.[10] Medical staff and the dominant medical model – which viewed the person in terms of physical systems, disease processes and treatment regimes – shaped nursing curricula. For some, nursing knowledge was a selection of facts and practice as tasks to be learned.[12] For others, it extended to include health and the patient's context, as in a 1923 syllabus that included medical knowledge (disease and treatment), concepts of health (the general rules of health) and institutional culture (patterns of ward work).[11] This developed to reflect a broadening in the scope of the knowledge that nurses needed. In 1959, for example, nurses' knowledge included *'hygiene, anatomy, physiology, chemistry, physics, pharmacy and psychotherapy'*.[13] A dominant medical view persisted well into the 1980s, with some nursing texts[14] continuing to espouse a physician-centric view of nursing practice.

Nurses' work was limited to their defined scope of practice (sick-room management or its later equivalent), and they were not to encroach on medical decision making or *'usurp the role of the medical man'*[9] by attempting to diagnose, prescribe or give an opinion on a case.[11] They were *'not expected to take on any responsibility outside their own sphere of work'*[15] or to *'act on her* (sic) *own responsibility except in an emergency'*.

Rules and decision making

The organisational context in those early days also established some patterns that persisted well into the later decades of the twentieth century. Each hospital had a series of local rules (known as hospital etiquette)[9] that nurses observed. Within this culture, nurses developed additional rules (*'compelled by experience'*) to secure decision outcomes of *'proper care for patients'*. This was seen as the mark of a good nurse, and rule-driven practice demonstrated compliance with the medical and organisational context. Obedience to hospital rules also lent support to the positional power of doctors in service delivery. Conformity was the rule of the day as nurses *'work(ed) under the doctor'* and ward sisters policed this by being *'responsible for the proper carrying out of all the duties and for the observance of order and discipline'.*[9] The potency of such socialisation into non-questioning obedience to doctors was commented on as a *'common experience that the more highly qualified is the nurse the less likelihood is there of her attempting to usurp the role of the medical man'.*[9] Some nurses colluded with these extrinsic views of their role[16] which depicted them as *'an aid in managing the sick'*, and went so far as to claim that any challenge brought *'discredit'* on themselves and their profession. Successful nursing practice was demonstrated by those *'who had learnt not to challenge doctors'*. This has been retrospectively likened to a family metaphor of domestic role divisions.[8] Where did it leave decision making? Nurses tended towards being medical assistants, provided information for doctors' decision making and followed rules as far as the legitimate scope of their decision making was concerned. How then could nurses' participation in decision making be described within a hierarchical and patriarchal care system?

Assistants in medical decision making

Nurses' work included information seeking and processing – observation, judgement, reporting and recording. Doctors regarded patient observation as the *'key function'* and *'the most helpful role that a nurse performed'.*[17] Observation had long been valued by doctors on account of nurses being with patients for longer than doctors. Even in the 1930s, observations were categorised as 'proper' and included appearance, behaviour, bodily systems and communication.[16] Current professional guidance still includes similar remarks about 'relevant' information.

Observations were made to identify change, implying information processing, which was reported to the doctor so that *'he may be enabled to make his diagnosis and orders regarding treatment'.*[18] Information processing also included descriptions of the type of change (e.g. *'sudden or insidious'*) but had to report not *'opinion but the facts observed by her* [the nurse] *during her period of duty'.* [18] Other doctors differed from this and wanted nurses to use *'an intelligent mind trained to observe and deduce'* and to avoid *'thinking on routine lines.'*[19]

Nurses were originally expected to report their observations to doctors verbally from memory, so that they could *'answer any questions about the conduct or appearance of her patient'*,[18] but increasingly used supplementary notes which were considered to be *'more handy and reliable than many memories'*. A formal nursing record was used as a communication book between doctors and nurses, and this contained medical orders, nurses' observations and nurses' notes of treatment given.[11,18]

Deciding what to report to a doctor represented one type of nurse decision, and implied learning what and when to report. Knowing how to do this was commonly described as *'an issue that required time and experience'.*[10] Some knowledge could be acquired in the classroom, but it would seem that its application in making decisions was learned in practice.

Breakout: developing nurse decision making

The scope of nurses has altered in the last 25 years, due to the combined effect of intrinsic and extrinsic factors. Nurses have sought to develop a nursing knowledge base and nursing diagnoses related to nursing therapy rather than medical treatment. In the 1950s and 1960s, nursing was rooted in a medically orientated *'emphasis upon fact, objectivity and reductionism'*, and the adoption of positivist approaches emulated the dominance of medical science and a medical model. Non-positivist methods were used to challenge existing patriarchal and *'class-based expositions of nursing'*.[20] Descriptions of nursing practice as an art and a science encompassed these differences.[13,21] Nurses' former practices of apprenticeship alongside an experienced nurse (learning the art of nursing) were challenged[22] as being insufficient to satisfy the contemporary need for a clear theoretical base, as this only perpetuated existing practices, whereas development of a theory base would enable practitioners to *'develop their own skills'*. However, with regard to learning the art of decision making there was limited evidence of teaching strategies that *'would be most beneficial to the development of decision-making skills in nursing'*.[23] The changing nature of nursing work has led some to conclude that *'it may never be possible to define the nursing contribution to patient care, due to the ever changing nature of this work'*.[24] The art–science dualism at least highlighted the need to acknowledge the use of different types of evidence in nurses' decision making.

Nursing models and decision making

Nursing is also expressed through the way in which nurses conceptualise their patients. The development of nursing models marked a departure from the dominant medical model and challenged it. In contrast to the biomedical gaze that focused on the body, cells and pathology, nurses in the 1960s and 1970s began to study other disciplines, developed conceptual systems of nursing and articulated grand theories.[25] The use of these marked a move from a doctor-led, task-orientated culture (with 'nursing orders' which persisted into the 1980s) towards a care-planning and problem-solving approach to care (also called the nursing process). It also marked a subtle change in purpose from helping the doctor to helping the patient.

A problem-solving approach to care had been sanctioned in 1977 by the General Nursing Council (UK). It led to the introduction of nursing diagnosis into UK practice that represented *'initial efforts to identify the phenomena that are of concern to nursing'*,[26] involving a *'clear nursing diagnosis and concept of the nursing problem'*.

An Activities of Daily Living (ADL) model of nursing was developed in 1980[21] and was claimed to be the first attempt by UK nurses to develop a conceptual model for nursing.[20] It has since become widely accepted in practice. Baroness McFarlane recorded the change that had been occurring in nursing from ritual-ised and institutional approaches to those that are rationally planned and individualised. She noted how Roper, Logan and Tierney[21] had defined the nurse in terms of elements of practice relating to the patient's functional ability. The preface of Roper, Logan and Tierney's' book[21] implied how a decision-making process utilised a core of knowledge that was augmented by experience, combined with specialised knowledge to develop a way of thinking about nursing to achieve stated outcomes (*'effective and compassionate nursing'*) in a range of contexts (*'people of whatever age who have various problems who are in different healthcare settings'*). Although assessment and intervention are stages of a prob-lem-solving process (assess, plan, implement and evaluate), this model did not explain how intervention decisions were made. However, it was a valuable step in crafting a definition of nursing practice, and it linked the art (experience) and science (process) of nursing practice.

So far it can be seen that decision making involves individuals who within the framework of a problem-solving approach make decisions by seeking and processing information. This is influenced by their method of conceptualising the patient (nursing model), and is informed by different types of *'knowledge from nursing and a variety of other disciplines as a basis for making nursing practice decisions'*.[27] Knowledge alone is insufficient to make decisions; clinically derived experience of using it is also necessary. A shift in practice has occurred that has strengthened independent decision making by nurses, but has not fully achieved autonomous decision-making status. The making of decisions requires skill, and some see the need for *'clinicians who are autonomous decision makers . . . [to] . . . develop effective problem-solving and decision-making skills'*.[28] This brief description of selected developments in describing nurses' decision making from sick-room managers to semi-autonomous problem-solving practitioners involves a decision maker, a decision process, a decision outcome and a decision context. The scope of nurses' legitimate decision making can be understood as being defined by the boundary established between the interplay of intrinsic and extrinsic factors (e.g. nursing development, policy shifts, medical dominance, views of the role of women as nurses).

Decision-making enquiry about different types of nurse

Nurses cannot be described as a homogenous group, but rather as several subgroups within a wider community. The decision-making practice of many of these subgroups has been examined. This has included coronary care nurses,[29] emergency nurses,[30] critical care nurses,[31,32] obstetric nurses,[33] neonatal nurses,[34] perioperative nurses,[35] general practice nurses,[2] advanced practice nurses,[36] expert nurses and midwives,[37] health visitors,[38] community nurses[39] and general nurses.[40]

Decision-making enquiry about different types of decision

A range of different types of nursing decision has been examined. These have included placing a person into residential care,[41] deciding when to call for emergency assistance,[42] intensive care unit nurses' transfer decisions,[43] triage decisions[44] and nurse prescribing.[45] Others have categorised the types of decision that nurses make – for example, intervention, communication and evaluation, and a further distinction between new and old decisions.[31]

Decision-making enquiry about process

The scope of nurse decision-making enquiry has included decision-maker relationships,[46] roles and identity as decision makers,[47,48] accountability,[49] decision outcomes[50] and explanations of practice errors.[51] An existing difficulty in nurse decision-making enquiry is the lack of consensus over a precise[52] and agreed use of terminology that has led to claims that decision-making studies *'may not even be reporting the same phenomenon'*.[53]

Decision-making enquiry and the use of different terminology

A range of terms has been used in reports on decision-making enquiry. These have included a reasoning process,[54] judgement,[55] reasoning strategies,[2] analytical and intuitive processes,[22,56] critical thinking[57] and discriminative thinking.[57] Terms such as decision making, problem solving, critical thinking, diagnostic reasoning and judgement are sometimes used interchangeably and their meaning requires clarification. Steps have been taken to classify nursing terminology, with several examples in use in the USA.[58,59] These are the North American Nursing Diagnosis Association (NANDA), the Nursing Interventions Classification (NIC), the Nursing Outcomes Classification (NOC), the Omaha System, the Georgetown University Home Healthcare Classification (HHCC), the Ozboldt partnership with the University Hospital Consortium (UHC) and the International Classification for Nursing Practice (ICNP).

Agreement in this area would offer a level of confidence that researchers were actually examining the same phenomenon across nursing subgroups. Its absence has been thought to impede the development and validation of standards to evaluate nursing practice, and is seen as an essential step in developing the role of the professional nurse. Other advantages that can be gained through agreeing a precise decision-making terminology include enhancing the visibility of nurses' contributions to healthcare delivery, and avoiding this being subsumed under the larger medical model.[49] The terms 'problem solving' and 'decision making' have been used synonymously,[60] and will be considered next.

Decision making and problem solving

Problem solving as a process has widespread agreement among nurses[61] and gives decision making a solution- or product-orientated focus.[62] However, problem-solving terminology is ill defined as *'unique'*,[37] *'reasoning'*[63] and *'dynamic'*.[64] Although it has been equated to the four-stage nursing process of assessment, planning, implementation and evaluation,[65] this has been challenged[66] to make the distinction that the nursing process was a tool used to plan care, whereas problem solving was a life skill. Descriptions of problem-solving steps (several,[67] three,[68] five[31] and six[2]) share common features of problem information, identification, interpretation and solution generation, and add clarity to approaches designed to facilitate learning the skill.

Decision-making outcomes

Problem solving and decision making both point to outcomes. These have been described in broad terms as to *'promote, maintain or regain health'*.[69] A scope of outcomes can be described, ranging from medical interests concerned with the detection and treatment of health disorders[70] to a health rather than illness focus,[71] or further towards a holistic stance, such as influencing a patient's well-being.[72] Other types of outcome can be categorised as being right for the patient[73] and appropriate.[2,47] Appropriateness can also refer to the process used by the nurse, such as *'discriminative thinking that led to the choice of a particular course of action'*[61] or *'the right course of action'*.[54] To understand what the right course of action may be and identify decision-making skills, it is useful to know how decision making has been theoretically explained. Two perspectives dominate decision-making explanations. These are prescriptive (also termed normative or rational) and descriptive (also termed intuitive or phenomenological) explanations.

Decision-making process: theoretical explanations

Descriptive and prescriptive explanations address different issues and use different methodologies. Prescriptive explanations are concerned with how decisions ought to be made and have an outcome focus.[74] They assume that the individual is a rational thinker and that human behaviour is logical and consistent. When making decisions, rational thought precedes action and is able to be made explicit. Decision trees and line-of-reasoning diagrams are typical ways of representing prescriptive decision making. These representations incorporate probability calculations and reduce the complexity of decision making to a series of variables and probabilities of outcomes.

In contrast, descriptive approaches are based on the assumption that action precedes rational thought, and correspond to a holistic view of nursing practice in which the decision maker sees the whole situation rather than reducing it to discrete elements. Descriptive explanations are concerned with how decisions are made, and focus on the processes involved. A unifying theory of decision making does not exist, although attempts have been made to develop one.[74]

The context of decision making: the clinical landscape

Nurses' decision making (in the UK) has developed since the 1800s from a medical assistant role that initially majored on sick-room management within a rule-driven and patriarchal context. It is accepted that nurses' roles include decision-making responsibility,[75] and that they make practice-orientated decisions which largely fall within two domains, namely nursing and medicine.[76] The patient links these, although some argue that doctors' *'traditional positional dominance'* remains.[46] A decision-making context continues to exist that includes the healthcare organisation and participants within a wider legal and social interpretation of nurses' roles. The term 'clinical landscape' has been used to describe this context.[77]

The changing technological context has contributed to nurses caring for more acutely ill patients using complex technology.[78] This has contributed to organisational change in efforts to make services more effective and efficient, and has run the risk of undervaluing knowing the patient in favour of prioritising *'organisational arrangements, economic restraints and efficiency of healthcare systems'*.[79]

Protocols and guidelines are a means of standardising approaches to decision making. Guidelines are *'systematically developed statements to assist practitioner and patient decisions about appropriate health care for specific clinical circumstances'*, [80] and comprise elements that describe different aspects of the patient's condition and the care to be given. They can form benchmarks for best practice, so are useful to healthcare organisations. A protocol is an explicit framework for the process of care, and members of the care team can follow precise steps of practice. Claims that these can aid nurses' decision making make assumptions about the nature of the evidence used in decision making and the 'correct' way of processing some information (e.g. investigations and observations).

Healthcare policy also shapes the clinical landscape. For example, the *'ruthless standardisation'*[81] required in the implementation of the NHS Plan[82] through the use of information technology claims to support clinical decision making so that *'those who give and receive care have the right information, at the right time'*.[71] Computer decision-support systems make specialist (expert) knowledge more widely available,[76] support nursing diagnosis and so are claimed to be an intelligent assistant and a valuable resource.

Human as well as non-human factors (e.g. patient situation, available resources and interpersonal relationships) shape the clinical landscape.[77] This landscape includes the nurse's *'duties, rights and social values'*.[83] Changes in the clinical landscape have also included developments in information and knowledge bases,[78] and implicate nurses as active participants through *'analysis, cue interpretation, [and] weighing evidence'*.[34] Descriptive decision-making processing terms, such as a *'gut feeling'*,[42] suggest links between the nurse, their experience, information and the generating of knowledge about a patient. Such individual factors in the clinical landscape are difficult to quantify and have resulted in claims that decision making was an *'unpredictable process'* and subject to *'changing practical exigencies'* of the context.[34] Clearly, more research is needed into the way in which these factors impact on decision making.[77]

The individual nurse as a factor in the clinical landscape gives rise to several questions. Much of their decision-making work is cognitive, and there is a need to make 'public' their narratives to describe the knowledge that is embedded in their practice and knowledge of patients. It has been argued that qualitative approaches to enquiry are useful[84] for making *'non-objective and less quantifiable clinical judgements visible and demonstrable'* and for uncovering knowledge that is embedded in practice.[85] The way in which nurses think has been associated with different types of decision maker. Novice decision makers have been described as deliberative, whereas experts think intuitively.[86] This raises the question of whether or not it is possible to think like an expert and learn by copying experts. It is questionable whether this can be achieved without identifying the essential elements of expert practice (e.g. practice-based knowledge), and in turn implies that the essential elements of a decision process can be known and made amenable to manipulation. Furthermore, it implies that there is an expert state of 'correct thinking', and it has long been acknowledged that expert decision making needs to be defined if these questions are to be answered.[37]

A bridge between novice and expert decision making was formed by applying context-free rules to guide action to being able to make a response that was intuitive or that came *'apparently out of nowhere'*.[87] This challenges other views that intuitive thinking was just a faster unconscious performance of analytic thinking processes, rather than a different form of thinking.[4] However, uncovering the nature of intuition as the defining factor in expertise is problematic, especially as intuitive judgement has been described as *'understanding without a rationale'*.[88] The types and processes of thinking, the participants, the context and the outcomes are all a part of decision making, and are shaped by the context in which the decision is made.

Conclusion

A nurse's role includes decision making that involves participants, process and outcomes, and which occurs in a given context. The context is shaped by many factors, human and non-human. It follows that decision making is contextually shaped, as are the scope and practice of nurses as decision makers. The two scenarios that were introduced at the beginning of this chapter can now be revisited to consider what needs to be asked about the decisions that nurses make. These questions must go beyond what happened (a particular intervention was carried out) to how and why a point of action was reached. This must include understanding how knowledge of the patient was constructed and shaped so that their problems or needs could be identified. The next chapter explores a decision-making model that centres on constructing an account of the patient, called a narrative. This model will be used to show how answers can be offered to questions of decision-making role, context and expertise.

Chapter summary box

- Nurses' roles as clinical decision makers are shaped by intrinsic and extrinsic factors.
- The clinical landscape describes the context of their decision making.
- Decision making includes a range of terms, some of which are used interchangeably.
- A precise definition of decision making does not exist.
- A unifying theory of nurses' decision making does not exist.
- There are different types of nursing decision.
- There are different types of nurse decision maker.
- There are different views on the thinking processes that are used when making decisions.
- The medical profession has dominated the development of nursing practice and therefore the scope of nurses' decision making.

Stop and think

This chapter has set the scene for further examination of decision making. Use the following questions as prompts for developing insights into decision-making enquiry that are directly related to the type of nursing work that is involved in your area of interest or work.

Origins

- If you had to describe the development of nurse decision making, which origin point would you select and why is this significant?
- Search out historical accounts of nursing practice. Sort them into time periods and abstract the direct or indirect remarks made about nurses' decision making.

- What points do they make about the process of decision making?
- What points do they make about the types and outcomes of decisions?
- What is the extent of nurses' decision authority?
- How have descriptions of nurses' decision making altered over the time period chosen?
- If the descriptions of decision making have altered, what reasons can you offer for this? Are these linked to policy, economics and social change?

Sub-area of nursing practice

- What aspects of practice have been examined in your chosen area of clinical nursing?
- Has the focus of decision-making enquiry within this practice altered over time?
- If so, are there any indications why the focus of enquiry has altered?

The elements of decision making

- Think about how you make decisions.
- Describe the process that you use.
- How would you explain your thinking to a trainee nurse as you make a decision?
- What is the legitimate scope of your decision making?
- Who has the authority to veto your decisions?

The clinical landscape

- Examine the clinical landscape in your chosen area of practice. What do you identify as the key features of the clinical landscape in the following areas:
  - organisational structures and practices
  - different staff groups
  - healthcare policies
  - technological advances?
- How do these shape nurses' work?
- When a clinical incident occurs, how is it investigated?
- What types of question are asked?
- To what extent do these generate explanations of how and why decisions are made?

References

1 These incidents actually occurred.
2 Offredy M (1998) The application of decision-making concepts by nurse practitioners in general practice. *J Adv Nurs.* **28**: 988–1000.
3 Corcoran SA (1986) Decision analysis: a step-by-step guide to making clinical decisions. *Nurs Healthcare.* **7**: 149–54.
4 Jones J (1988) Clinical reasoning in nursing. *J Adv Nurs.* **13**: 185–92.
5 Buckingham CD and Adams A (2000) Classifying clinical decision making: interpreting nursing intuition, heuristics and medical diagnosis. *J Adv Nurs.* **32**: 990–98.
6 Nightingale F (1859) *Notes on Nursing. What it is, and what it is not.* Churchill Livingstone, Edinburgh.
7 Stapleton M (1983) *Ward Sisters: another perspective.* Royal College of Nursing, London.
8 Hardey M (1998) *The Social Context of Health.* Open University Press, Buckingham.
9 Watson JK (1925) *A Handbook for Nurses* (5e). Scientific Press Ltd, London.
10 Pierce B (ed.) (1923) *Handbook for Mental Nurses* (7e). Ballière Tindall and Cox, London.
11 Henderson J (1921) *Medicine for Nurses.* Edward Arnold, London.
12 Pearn OPN (1936) *Mental Nursing (Simplified)* (2e). Ballière Tindall and Cox, London.
13 Pavey AE (1959) *The Story of the Growth of Nursing as an Art, a Vocation and a Profession* (5e). Faber and Faber, London.
14 Bloom A and Bloom S (1984) *Toohey's Medicine for Nurses* (14e). Churchill Livingstone, Edinburgh.
15 Scott DH and Hainsworth M (1936) *Modern Professional Nursing. Volume 2.* Caxton Publishing Co. Ltd, London.
16 Cahusac AN, Audland WE, Duncan RB, Lakin AT and Modlin IG (1932) *Home Nursing.* St John Ambulance Association, London.
17 Ashdown M (1925) *A Complete System of Nursing* (6e). JM Dent and Sons Ltd, New York.
18 Hainsworth M (ed.) (1949) *Modern Professional Nursing. Volume 2.* Caxton Publishing Co. Ltd, London.
19 Hitch M (1943) *Aids to Medicine for Nurses* (2e). Ballière Tindall, London.
20 Berragan E (1998) Nursing practice draws upon several ways of knowing. *J Clin Nurs.* **7**: 209–17.
21 Roper N, Logan WL and Tierney AJ (1980) *The Elements of Nursing.* Churchill Livingstone, Edinburgh.
22 Harbison J (1991) Clinical decision making in nursing. *J Adv Nurs.* **16**: 404–7.
23 Ellis PA (1987) Processes used by nurses to make decisions in the clinical practice setting. *Nurse Educ Today.* **17**: 325–32.
24 Spilsbury K and Meyer J (2001) Defining the nursing contribution to patient outcome: lessons from a review of the literature examining nursing outcomes, skill mix and changing roles. *J Clin Nurs.* **10**: 3–14.
25 Pearson A (1992) Knowing nursing: emerging paradigms in nursing. In: K Robinson and B Vaughan (eds) *Knowledge for Nursing Practice.* Butterworth-Heinemann, Oxford.
26 Hogston R (1997) Nursing diagnosis and classification systems: a position paper. *J Adv Nurs.* **26**: 496–500.
27 Valiga T (1983) Cognitive development: a critical component of baccalaureate education. *Image J Nurs Sch.* **15**: 115–19.
28 Boney J and Baker JD (1997) Strategies for teaching clinical decision making. *Nurse Educ Today.* **17**: 16–21.
29 Corcoran-Perry SA, Narayan SM and Cochrane S (1999) Coronary care nurses' clinical decision making. *Nurs Health Sci.* **1**: 49–61.
30 Lyneham J (1998) The process of decision making by emergency nurses. *Aust J Adv Nurs.* **16**: 7–14.

31 Bucknall T (2000) Critical care nurses' decision-making activities in the natural clinical setting. *J Clin Nurs.* **9**: 25–36.

32 Aitken LM (2003) Critical care nurses' use of decision-making strategies. *J Clin Nurs.* **12**: 476–83.

33 Haggerty LA and Nuttall RL (2000) Experienced obstetric nurses' decision making in fetal risk situations. *J Obstet Gynecol Neonatal Nurs.* **29**: 489–90.

34 Greenwood J, Sullivan J, Spence K and McDonald M (2000) Nursing scripts and the organizational influences on critical thinking: a report of a study of neonatal nurses' clinical reasoning. *J Adv Nurs.* **31**: 106–14.

35 Parker CB, Minick P and Kee C (1999) Clinical decision-making processes in perioperative nursing. *AORN J.* **70**: 45–62.

36 Lipman HT and Deatrick AJ (1997) Preparing advanced practice nurses for clinical decision making in speciality practice. *Nurse Educator.* **22**: 47–50.

37 Orme L and Maggs C (1993) Decision making in clinical practice: how do expert nurses, midwives and health visitors make decisions? *Nurse Educ Today.* **13**: 270–76.

38 Lemmer B (1998) Successive surveys of an expert panel: research in decision making with health visitors. *J Adv Nurs.* **27**: 538–45.

39 Bryans A. and MacIntosh J (1996) Decision making in community nursing: an analysis of the stages of decision making as they relate to community nursing assessment practice. *J Adv Nurs.* **24**: 24–30.

40 Lamond D, Crow R, Chase J, Doggen K and Swinkels M (1996) Information sources used in decision making: considerations for simulation development. *Int J Nurs Stud.* **33**: 47–57.

41 Armstrong M (2000) Factors affecting the decision to place a relative with dementia into residential care. *Nurs Standard.* **14**: 33–7.

42 Cioffi J (2000) Nurses' experience of making decisions to call emergency assistance to their patients. *J Adv Nurs.* **31**: 108–14.

43 Higgins LW (1999) Nurses' perceptions of collaborative nurse–physician transfer decision making as a predictor of patient outcomes in a medical intensive care unit. *J Adv Nurs.* **29**: 1434–43.

44 Cone KJ and Murray R (2000) Characteristics, insights, decision making and preparation of ED triage nurses. *J Emerg Nurs.* **28**: 401–6.

45 Luker K, Hogg C, Austin I, Fergusson B and Smith K (1998) Decision making: the context of prescribing. *J Adv Nurs.* **27**: 657–65.

46 Trede F and Higgs J (2003) Re-framing the clinician's role in collaborative decision making: re-thinking practice knowledge and the notion of clinician–patient relationships. *Learn Health Soc Care.* **2**: 66–73.

47 Joseph DH (1985) Sex role stereotype, self-concept, education and experience: do they influence decision making? *Int J Nurs Stud.* **22**: 21–32.

48 Rhodes BA (1985) Occupational ideology and clinical decision making in British nursing. *Int J Nurs Stud.* **22**: 241–57.

49 Maas ML (1998) Advancing nursing's accountability for outcomes. *Outcomes Management for Nursing Practice.* **1** (1): 3–4.

50 Maas ML, Delaney C and Huber D (1999) Contextual variables and assessment of the outcome effects of nursing interventions. *Outcomes Management for Nursing Practice.* **3** (1): 4–6.

51 Meurier CE, Vincent CA and Parmer DG (1998) Nurses' responses to severity-dependent errors: a study of the causal attributions made by nurses following an error. *J Adv Nurs.* **27**: 349–54.

52 Thompson C and Dowding D (eds) (2002) *Clinical Decision Making and Judgement in Nursing.* Churchill Livingstone, London.

53 Thompson C, McCaughan D, Cullum N, Sheldon TA, Mulhall A and Thompson DR

(2001) Research information in nurses' clinical decision making: what is useful? *J Adv Nurs.* **36**: 376–88.

54 Karlsson S, Bucht G, Rasmussen B and Sandman PO (2000) Restraint in elder care: decision making among registered nurses. *J Clin Nurs.* **9**: 842–50.

55 Cioffi J (1997) Heuristics, servants to intuition, in clinical decision making. *J Adv Nurs.* **26**: 203–8.

56 King L and Appleton JV (1997) Intuition: a critical review of the research and rhetoric. *J Adv Nurs.* **26**: 194–202.

57 Lipman M (1988) Critical thinking: what can it be? *Anal Teaching.* **8**: 5–12.

58 Keenan G and Aquilino ML (1998) Standardized nomenclatures: keys to continuity of care, nursing accountability and clinical effectiveness. *Outcomes Manag Nurs Pract.* **2 (2)**: 81–6.

59 Moen A, Henry S and Warren J (1999) Representing nursing judgements in the electronic health record. *J Adv Nurs.* **30**: 990–97.

60 Lamond D, Crow R and Chase J (1996) Judgements and processes in care decisions in acute medical and surgical wards. *J Eval Clin Pract.* **2**: 211–16.

61 Moore P (1996) Decision making in professional practice. *Br J Nurs.* **5**: 635–40.

62 Duchscher JEB (1999) Catching the wave: understanding the concept of critical thinking. *J Adv Nurs.* **29**: 577–83.

63 Baker JD (1997) Phenomenography: an alternative approach to researching the clinical decision making of nurses. *Nurs Inquiry.* **4**: 41–7.

64 Marsden J (1998) Decision making in A&E by expert nurses. *Nurs Times.* **94**: 62–5.

65 Chang AM and Gaskill D (1991) Nurses' perceptions of their problem-solving ability. *J Adv Nurs.* **16**: 813–19.

66 Taylor C (1997) Problem solving in clinical nursing practice. *J Adv Nurs.* **26**: 329–36.

67 Schaefer J (1974) The interrelatedness of the decision-making process and the nursing process. *Am J Nurs.* **74**: 1852–5.

68 Jones RAP and Beck SE (eds) (1996) *Decision Making in Nursing.* Delmar Publishers, London.

69 Grossman CC and Hudson DB (2001) Rating students' technology-generated clinical decision-making scores. *Nurse Educ.* **26 (1)**: 5, 12.

70 Bradshaw A (2000) Competence and British nursing: a view from history. *J Clin Nurs.* **9**: 321–9.

71 Woolley N (1991) An expert to help you give the right care. Expert systems in clinical decision making. *Prof Nurse.* **May:** 431–6.

72 Bulmer C (1998) Clinical decisions: defining meaning through focus groups. *Nurs Standard.* **12**: 12, 20, 34–6.

73 Panniers TL and Walker EK (1994) A decision-analytic approach to clinical nursing. *Nurs Res.* **43**: 245–9.

74 Buckingham CD and Adams A (2000) Classifying clinical decision making: a unifying approach. *J Adv Nurs.* **32**: 981–9.

75 Simpson E and Courtney M (2002) Critical thinking in nursing education: literature review. *Int J Nurs Pract.* **8**: 89–98.

76 Hedberg B and Larsson US (2002) Observations, conformations and strategies – useful tools in decision-making process for nurses in practice? *J Clin Nurs.* **12**: 215–22.

77 Bucknall T (2003) The clinical landscape of critical care: nurses' decision making. *J Adv Nurs.* **43**: 310–19.

78 Profetto-McGrath J (2003) The relationship of critical thinking dispositions of baccalaureate nursing students. *J Adv Nurs.* **43**: 569–77.

79 Whittemore R (2000) Consequences of not 'knowing the patient.' *Clin Nurse Specialist.* **14**: 75–81.

80 Fennessy G (1998) Guidelines and protocols. *Pract Nurs.* **9**: 14–16.

81 Department of Health (2000) *A Health Service of all the Talents: developing the NHS workforce*. Department of Health, London.

82 www.npfit.nhs.uk

83 Corcoran SA (1986) Task complexity and nursing expertise as factors in decision making. *Nurs Res.* **35:** 107–12.

84 Benner P and Wrubel J (1982) Skilled clinical knowledge: the value of perceptual awareness. *Nurse Educator.* **May/June:** 11–17.

85 Tanner CA, Benner P, Chesla C and Gordon DR (1993) The phenomenology of knowing the patient. *Image J Nurs Sch.* **25:** 273–80.

86 Benner P (1984) *From Novice to Expert: power and excellence in nursing practice*. Addison and Wesley, Menlow Park, California.

87 Rolfe G (1997) Science, abduction and the fuzzy nurse: an exploration of expertise. *J Adv Nurs.* **25:** 1070–75.

88 Benner P and Tanner C (1987) How expert nurses use intuition. *Am J Nurs.* **87:** 22–31.

Chapter 2

Making clinical decisions: a model of nurses' decision making

Introduction

A model of nurses' clinical decision making is described in this chapter and will be referred to in subsequent chapters. The model represents how nurses construct knowledge of their patients. I have labelled this as the development of a narrative about a patient, which is the story or account that expresses how the patient is known. Narrative development has a cyclic characteristic, but for clarity of explanation I shall describe its different stages in a linear manner. In this way I shall describe how a fleeting account about a patient is developed into a narrative that is shared by a team of nurses and individually owned by each one of them. Nurses use their narrative to identify the patient's needs and to select corresponding interventions. A decision is made when an intervention (or more than one) has been chosen. A brief overview of the narrative follows, before I move on to examine its stages of development in more detail. Figure 2.1 illustrates the stages of narrative development as part of nurses' clinical decision making.

An overview of narrative development

Narrative development commences with a pre-admission account about a patient that is developed into an admission account following the patient's arrival on the ward. Successive revisions through information seeking and processing at individual and team levels support the transformation of the narrative from a story about knowing the patient to one that is owned by the nurse who can claim to 'know' the patient. On the basis of knowing, the patient's needs are identified and interventions chosen. Clinical decision making therefore rests on how the patient is known.

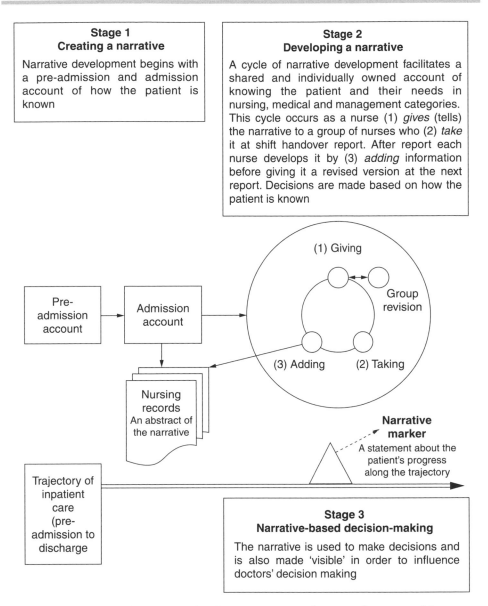

Figure 2.1 The stages of narrative development as part of nurses' decision making.

Stage 1: Pre-admission and admission stages

During the pre-admission and admission stages, information about the patient is initially received and subsequently used to seek more information to construct an account of them. This is shaped by the nurse's roles and how these direct enquiry for particular types of information. This is chiefly information in relation to caring, care management and medical domains. The focus of the nurse's information seeking can be described as using different lenses according to their different roles. I have collectively termed these a *conceptual lens*.

Stage 2: Report

Next the admission account is informally communicated to other nurses on duty, sometimes on a one-to-one basis. However, it is formally told, or 'given', during the next shift handover report to nurses commencing their shift. In report, nurses 'take' each narrative through listening and note taking. Note taking is part of a process of committing the narrative to memory. Often, narrative giving follows a sequence that includes references to the nursing record (called a Kardex) and also to nurses' personal note sheets. This process of information giving and taking is part of the development of a group consensus about how the patient is known. It often involves discussion in which the narrative is challenged, corroborated or revised by the team.

Written records were compiled contemporaneously, but the narratives contained in these differed from their verbal counterparts. This difference will be examined in Chapter 4 together with the informal temporary notes written by nurses.

Stage 3: Caregiving

After report, nurses proceeded to care for their patients, often without referring to written care records until the end of the shift. This created opportunities to check the existing narrative and add new information to it. In this way the individual nurse developed their own version of the narrative which was subsequently passed on to other nurses at the next report. A continuing cycle of narrative giving and taking, team review, individual checking and adding new information continued shift after shift, day after day. The construction of knowing the patient is therefore dynamic.

These three stages of narrative development – giving and taking, developing and giving to the next group of nurses – (*see* Figure 2.1) contribute to ongoing narrative development along the patient's journey through their experience of hospitalisation. I have called this journey their *trajectory of care* (*see* Figure 2.2), as a chronological journey extending from pre-admission, through admission, continuing care and treatment to the point of the patient being discharged from hospital. These narrative stages will now be examined further.

Pre-admission
Ward staff are notified about the patient and create a pre-admission account
⇩
Admission
Ward staff develop first-hand knowledge of the patient and develop an admission narrative
⇩
Continuing care period
Ward staff provide planned care and treatment with and for the patient. The narrative is continually revised
⇩
Discharge from hospital care
The patient exits from the programme of care and treatment. The narrative is ended and a record of it may contribute to a future pre-admission and admission narrative

Figure 2.2 The trajectory of care.

Narrative development stage 1: Pre-admission accounts and admission narratives

It's essentially looking for what is wrong with the patient and thinking ahead as to what needs to be done.

The pre-admission account

The pre-admission stage marks the beginning of a patient's journey along the care trajectory. It involves a ward nurse forming an initial impression about the patient before actually meeting them. The substance of this impression is drawn from secondary information sources, usually via a telephone conversation with whoever is referring the patient to the ward. This includes general practitioners, Accident and Emergency nurses or doctors and medical staff from other wards who are authorising a transfer of a patient from elsewhere in the hospital. Pre-admission information also includes excerpts from the patient's medical and nursing records. The nurse uses it to anticipate the patient's needs and prepare for their arrival on the ward.

In the following discussion, Julie, a staff nurse, explained how she developed her account of John, a patient who was being transferred from the Accident and Emergency department. She had been informed that *'The SHO (senior house officer) had telephoned through that a 43-year-old patient was coming who has a two-day history of coffee-ground vomiting.'* John's medical casenotes had already been delivered to the ward, and Julie skim-read them: *'He has had a number of previous admissions for epigastric pain – they (doctors) have been querying pancreatitis and that was followed up by a gastroscopy and triple drug therapy treatment. He had then not been taking all of the prescribed medication and also had defaulted from (hospital) appointments. He subsequently had an overdose, and had also not attended for a planned vasectomy.'*

Julie's account included medical history information (*'a number of previous admissions'*), diagnosis (*'epigastric pain . . . querying pancreatitis'*), previous investigation and treatment plans (*a gastroscopy and triple drug therapy'*), and John's compliance with this. She depicted John as a medical 'case' who was not compliant with a prescribed medical treatment plan. Given that her account lacked first-hand information derived from her own observations and discussion with John, I asked her how valid it was. She sounded a note of caution, stating that it was *'awful really, but you do form an impression'*. The problem is whether or not this impression is valid.

The validity of such accounts is strengthened when the nurse has previously cared for the patient. This allows a comparative judgement to be made between a previous and current admission to anticipate the patient's needs.

Sister Zoe, after taking a telephone referral from a GP, explained how previous knowledge of a patient did influence her pre-admission account. *'He was started on a drug which the GP prescribed, not the hospital, as it was quite expensive and a new drug. It sounds like he is having problems of reactions to it and will need to come in.'* Enquiring further about the reason for the admission, she replied that it was *'to wean him off the drug and for him to be reassessed. The doctor will need to review him by the sound of it . . . having said that, he might say the patient can be nursed at home! But I think that he will admit him. We know the patient.'*

As in the earlier account of John, this also included medical information ('*started on a drug*') and the patient's response ('*it sounds like he is having problems of reactions to it*'), but was triangulated with previous knowledge of nursing him ('*we know the patient*'). Sister Zoe processed this information to make a judgement about the patient's need for admission ('*will need to come in*'), linking this to medical needs ('*to wean him off the drug*' and '*to be reassessed*'), and anticipated the doctor's decision ('*I think that he will admit him*'). Prior knowledge of caring for this patient supported the nurse's confidence in her own pre-admission account and anticipation of needs.

Both accounts amount to little more than an impression that the nurses used to anticipate needs and make preparations for the patient's arrival on the ward. However, many nurses regarded pre-admission accounts as unreliable, as they were largely based on secondary information sources. These represented knowledge *about* the patient rather than *of* the patient. Tony, a charge nurse, explained how relying on these accounts led to inaccurate anticipation of needs and the making of inappropriate preparatory decisions. A contributing factor to the unreliability of pre-admission accounts was attributed to the referring nurse's lack of knowledge of a patient, and was summarised as '*staff* [who] *are moving patients on* [from another department] *who don't know them that well*'.

He continued, '*We get people sent up and they are said to be independent and don't need much care, only to assess their state on arrival to the ward as dependent and in need of nursing care. When they come they need about six staff to move them, or are moribund, and they get allocated to perhaps an inappropriate part of the ward because of the report given.*'

In this case, the pre-admission account was triangulated with one generated through direct observation, allowing a comparative judgement to be made about the patient's health and subsequent reassessment of their needs. At this stage of the process nurses did make decisions – preparatory ones while they were awaiting the patient's arrival on the ward.

Pre-admission account decisions

Decisions were made about the physical preparations needed to nurse the patient, and also about what to ask about during the patient assessment interview. Physical preparations included designating a particular bed, and preparing equipment such as monitors and infusion pumps. A part of this was not dissimilar to nurses' sick-room management of a previous era, in which they controlled the environment in which the patient was placed. However, the preparation for the assessment interview began to reveal how the nurse 'saw' the patient in relation to the pre-admission account, their role and understanding of the purpose of the admission phase.

Nurses described variations in their approach to information seeking during the admission, which included the use of a general questioning framework and a cue-driven approach. Some nurses described the general framework as '*a set patter which I ask – it's a bit like the police do when it comes to telling them about their property – but I tend to have the same sort of questions which I ask*'. A cue-driven approach picked up on statements in the pre-admission account. For example, a patient with 'alcohol problems' was going to be asked specifically about '*the alcohol intake and if he is still a heavy drinker, and about his medication at present.*'

Although these decisions might seem cursory with regard to the actual care that the patient subsequently received, and the pre-admission account did change, their importance lies in the glimpse that it offers into nurses' thinking. These decisions shaped how the narrative developed and became personally owned. The admission account moved this process on.

The admission account

Once the patient arrived on the ward, the pre-admission account began to be developed into an admission narrative. Information was gathered through observation and interview. During these interviews the reliability of the pre-admission account was checked and discrepancies identified: *'You ask patients if they have any past medical history, they tell you "no", and then you find that they have a laparotomy scar or something like that.'* Similarly, direct observation was sometimes sufficient to discount the reliability of a pre-admission account, as in the case of a patient who was expected to arrive at the ward *'in a wheelchair with a vomit bowl'* but in fact walked in and was not nauseous.

Medical records were sometimes seen as being more useful during the admission process than nursing records. A staff nurse explained how she favoured medical model information to establish the reason for the patient being on the ward and what their problems might be: *'I don't trust what another nurse tells me when we get a new patient. I look at the medical case notes. Sometimes there is hardly anything written on the nursing sheet when they come from the Medical Assessment Unit. No diagnosis or anything like that. Take this, for example. It said he had back pain and weight loss. I felt that he might have a malignancy because he is a heavy smoker. So I looked in the medical notes and found that they are querying some malignancy and are doing tests.'*

Sometimes nurses augmented their admission narrative with information from outside the ward – for example, by telephoning community nurses who had cared for the patient prior to the admission. *'If the patient has been living in a rest home I read the notes. I might ring the rest home to see what normal care for the patient was like. They* [rest home staff] *will give a verbal report of the patient's mobility and wheelchair use, etc., but their history doesn't get written in the rest home notes.'*

Information seeking was used to make comparative judgements between accounts of the patient's pre-admission and admission health status so that needs could be identified and a plan of care developed. Needs identification and planning revealed the nurse's purpose in the whole admission process, which was described as *'essentially looking for what is wrong with the patient and thinking ahead as to what needs to be done'*. A medical focus underpinned the meaning of *'what is wrong'*, and the nurse's role corresponded to understanding medical interventions: *'What's wrong – where is the patient's treatment going?'* The nurse's roles in relation to information seeking will be examined shortly, but first I shall consider what shaped information seeking.

Shaping information seeking

The nursing record was a popular tool used to shape nurses' information seeking. This record was divided into several sections corresponding to an Activities of

Daily Living model.[1] Each section was used as a prompt for questioning the patient:

> *I use the Roper model because I trained using that and have only worked here. I have a question list in my mind relating to each section of the form and I tend to go through the same questions with everyone. For example, with diet I ask if they are diabetic or have a special diet, whether or not they drink alcohol, and if so how much.*

The extent of the admission interview was limited by competing workload pressures, principally the care of other patients and associated clerical work. Time figured prominently in this (*'the time available and the other patients needing to be seen'*), and an admission interview varied from *'about 10 to 15 minutes, but was longer if investigations such as ECG monitoring* [electrocardiogram, a form of cardiac monitoring] *were required'*. Administration, particularly record keeping, was cited as doubling the total assessment workload to the extent that *'with all the paper and investigations it can take 45 minutes to an hour to complete'*. The requirement to compile contemporaneous records also meant that some nurses stayed beyond the end of their shift to complete their records.

Time management was clearly a factor in patient assessment discussions, and two strategies were used to manage this, namely short cuts and curtailing patient discussion. A short cut was used when the patient had a record of a previous admission to hospital. In these instances old information was copied from previous case notes and used to focus questioning. Unfortunately, this action led to a one-sided conversation in which the nurse aimed to *'just . . . verify a lot of previous details'*. Despite this, nurses claimed that they valued the patient's response as *'you can never be sure unless you check with the patient'*, but a short cut only modified a previous account through marginal revisions. Furthermore, the opportunity to explore other health issues that might have been of concern to the patient was limited. In defence of short cuts, nurses claimed that the amount of interaction taking place was down to the patient: *'it depends upon how much they want to talk to you'*. This was not necessarily the case, as some nurses curtailed a patient's conversation if it was delaying their completion of the assessment: *'It* [assessment] *can take minutes, but others talk and talk and you have to focus it.'* Focusing involved taking control of the discussion: *'He* [the patient] *talked and talked and I had to actually say that we needed to get on with the assessment.'*

It can be seen that information seeking was influenced by time, the purpose of the assessment and the approach taken by the nurse. Consequently, this introduced a degree of selectivity which left other areas of information unexplored. Selectivity in information seeking is also linked to the different roles that nurses adopted in the clinical setting. These directed the nurse's gaze in information seeking. Figure 2.3 shows how this gaze is represented as a lens that has three facets corresponding to the nurse's roles. Each facet is used to seek a specific type of information.

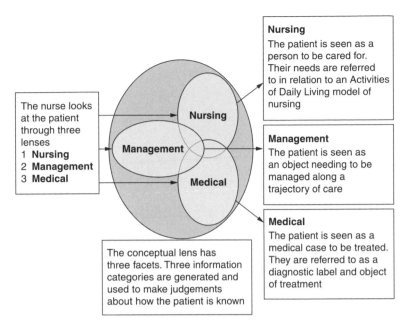

Figure 2.3 The three facets of the conceptual lens used by nurses in information seeking.

Role and information seeking: nurse as carer

The term 'nurse' encompasses several roles and cannot be assumed to be a homogenous single entity. These roles shaped their information seeking. A common role that was described as a core feature of nurses' work, regardless of grade – whether referring to themselves as a standard nurse, manager or advanced practitioner – was *'hands on'* or *'basic care.'* This was characterised by *'a good bedside manner'* and seen as a *'nursing priority'* that emphasised *'the important role of the nurse'*, which was being patient focused, chiefly *'looking after the sick.'* Nurses claimed that a basic care role was compatible with a holistic view of the patient that addressed his or her physical, social and psychological needs.

Ward managers took a broader role perspective than some junior nurses, which emphasised management concerns linked to their *'responsibility to know what is going on in the whole ward.'* They valued basic care as the *'traditional'* heritage of practice, and required other nurses to take a *'pride in ensuring that these tasks are completed.'* They also implied that threats to basic care delivery existed: *'Before I had a closer contact and would be thinking on how I would reduce the* [patient's] *discomfort. There was less time constraint. Now it is so busy and things get forgotten . . . as sister you have to keep more in your head and there is less time. It can be mentally exhausting.'*

These tasks of care had an enduring or traditional characteristic:

> *A traditional role, one where you give attention to detail, patients are fed and washed, are wearing appropriate clothing. Other things are important but you have to get the basics right first and the other comes with it. There needs to be pride in making sure that they're washed, clean and tidy, the medicines and dressings are done and the observations are done.*

These expressions of responses to needs identification by implication demonstrated that nurses were making numerous individualised decisions. The promotion of the nurse's role as carer thus encouraged engagement with knowing the patient and making care decisions: *'I try to instil that in everyone, it "narks"* [annoys] *me the most when the basics are not attended to.'* Clinical decision making included, but was not limited to, tasks representing the nurse as carer. Indeed some junior nurses were described by experienced staff as having a limited understanding of the patient, being described as *'task focused'*. This was corroborated by ward managers, who acknowledged that juniors were *'good at tasks'*. Although tasks represented a limited role perspective, attention to them was valuable, especially in relation to complaints, as these were often *'the thing we get the most complaints about'*.

Engagement in care tasks was also an opportunity to seek more information about them: *'Basic care is about being sure that the patient is comfortable and clean in a physical sense. It is also about ensuring that they are comfortable with where they are and are able to talk* [for example, asking], *"Sister, can I chat with you?", so that they can talk about their problems.'*

Information seeking through basic caregiving allowed the nurse to check that care was meeting a range of needs and to find out the patient's views about their illness and hospitalisation. This information was included in the developing narrative about the patient. Nurses used their knowledge of the patient with care needs to be an advocate for them. Advocacy was described as being a *'go-between – between the patients and doctors'* in which they acted as an *'interpreter for the patient'* to doctors. This, they argued, was necessary because *'doctors with the elderly don't understand what they* [patients] *are saying and they need someone to interpret across the culture'*. It was mentioned earlier that nurses' pre-admission accounts were closely linked with a medical view of the patient and, in being an advocate, the nurse had to decide how to represent the patient to the doctor. This process amounted to *'a matter of judgement'* according *'to the nurse as they stand by the patient'*. The interactions between nurses and doctors in making narratives known will be examined further in Chapter 5, as games nurses play. These games reveal how different ways of knowing the patient exist in the ward, and how the nurses' way of knowing (the narrative) can be used to alter the medical treatment plan. These interactions also made apparent the nurse's care management role.

Role and information seeking: nurse as care manager

Experienced nurses who discussed their care management role spoke of their *'ownership'* of care beyond *'more than just the work that staff nurses did'*. They recognised a need *'to organise the management of patients'* arising from their *'responsibility to know what is going on in the whole ward, somebody needs to see to that'*. Nurses' decisions as care managers encroached on the *'territory of the junior doctor'* due to concerns over ineffective medical case management. For example, some *'consultants did not know what their junior doctors had done regarding case management'*.

As care managers, sisters and experienced staff nurses saw themselves as a *'fulcrum'* at the interface between managing and delivering patient care. They regarded themselves in this role as an information hub, and nurses in general as more likely to have a broad scope of information about patients due to their 24-

hour presence on the ward. '*Everyone* [non-nurses] *who comes on to the ward is prescriptive, they just come and go, but the nurse is at the centre of things. They are always there, so they get it* [information] *from all directions.*'

They were also a focus for less-experienced team members who sought peer guidance via this information hierarchy. Sister Kath, a ward manager, explained:

> *The junior nurse is task focused. As far as the staff are concerned I am here as 'mother'. So I am a focus for them. They can go and ask the sister – she will probably know. I know who to go to to sort things out because I have worked here for so long. I know a lot of staff on surgery, and have seen many of them pass through as students. Usually I will know what to do, but if I don't I will know someone who might. You should have a rapport with other wards, especially if you want to transfer patients. The hospital has always been like that.*

Sister Kath retained an overview of patients' problems and acted as an information resource for other nurses. This included processing information brought by other nurses who approached her '*to sort out things*' as part of making or guiding their decision making. The use of the term 'mother' revealed a relational and hierarchical information-seeking structure that extended beyond the ward.

Patients and their relatives also saw the ward sister as a reference point for information, and would bypass staff nurses to ask her questions, even about minor issues such as details of ward visiting times. Other nurses recognised this and associated the symbolism of a sister's dark blue uniform with having a greater level of knowledge, even if this was not necessarily true: '*The patients perceive that a dark blue uniform means that you know more than someone in a white uniform.*' . . . '*A staff nurse can tell them the same information but the dark uniform seems to instil confidence.*'

A part of information seeking associated with the management of the patient along the care trajectory included medical information. This gave rise to a third role, namely the nurse as medical assistant. Care management involved coordinating the contribution to the healthcare team, especially doctors, who were frequently regarded as having a limited perspective of the patient beyond medical concerns:

> *For example, consultants – they are typically totally divorced from the reality of planning a discharge of a patient who went home and died. The doctors don't take into account the service arrangements involved. For example, on a Friday there is no support available. Doctors get very blinkered and make decisions without thinking of these things. All they think is that they have got a patient with a surgical or medical problem and have a thing to fix or make better, and once done they don't see why they can't go home there and then. When they decide they can't do any more for them they decide to discharge* [the patient] *without making any mention of it until then.*

Many but not all doctors were like this. Some '*doctors are better – they look at the patient and ask selves if they can manage at home. They ask "If we let you go home, will you cope?"*' A part of care management therefore involved nurses' resistance to doctors' unilateral decision making about patients: '*With junior doctors we tell them not to tell the patient that they can go home until we have discussed all the issues we need to deal with prior to discharge.*'

Role and information seeking: nurse as medical assistant

The prominent role of doctors in medical wards influenced nurses' work to the extent that they actively sought some medical information so that they could *'know – like the doctors'* – that is, have a medical perspective of the patient and their treatment needs. Whereas the nursing model that was used was thought to be holistic, it was recognised that *'The doctors all use a medical model and that works for them. The doctors need to know what is happening from their viewpoint and we obviously have to work alongside that.'*

Nurses who took on a medical assistant role were concerned with *'getting work done'* in the belief that junior doctors were *'too busy to do everything'* and needed help in *'completing blood investigation forms'* and *'changing drips'*. They sought information that supported medical diagnostic decision making, and typically described this work as follows: *'Well, we admit them before the doctor sees them. I did the admission paperwork, routine bloods, the ECG was already done, card for X-ray. Then I went to inform the doctor who was on the unit about the findings, the admission to date. He will then go and see her and make a provisional diagnosis and decide what to prescribe as current treatment.'*

Such work could involve following routines, as acknowledged in *'we take too much blood'*, indicating that the rationale behind this was unclear. Nurses also described medical knowledge as being useful so that they could *'be sure of our knowledge about practice'*, and at times supported an information-seeking focus that was *'more medically orientated than on other wards'*. Indeed, medical knowledge was favoured over that found in the nursing record. During the admission phase, for example, a staff nurse commented that *'I don't trust what another nurse tells me, when we get a new patient I look at the medical case notes.'* Diagnostic information was particularly sought: *'Sometimes there is hardly anything written on the nursing sheet when they come from the medical assessment unit. No diagnosis or anything like that. Take this, for example* [selecting a nursing record], *it said he had back pain and weight loss. I felt that he might have a malignancy because he is a heavy smoker. So I looked in the medical notes and found that they* [doctors] *are querying some malignancy and are doing tests.'* Nurses' emphasis on a medical assistant role often rendered nursing care and nursing care decisions invisible, these being addressed *'on an as-required basis'*, and by implication many were not recorded.

Role and information seeking: a summary

Nurses' roles in wards (nurse as carer, care manager and medical assistant) are associated with three types of information seeking. These three roles help to describe the meaning of the term *medical ward nurse*.* As mentioned previously, information gathering can be explained as the nurse using a conceptual lens that has three facets corresponding to their roles (*see* Figure 2.3). They 'see' the patient through this to generate three information categories. They then process the latter to develop knowledge of the patient and use this to represent how the patient is known. It follows that a preference for one lens facet over others shapes

---

* A ward nurse in this study can be defined as a registered person whose role is to provide patient-centred care, managing the patient along a trajectory of care while coordinating the contributions of a multi-disciplinary team.

the emphasis that is given to how the patient is known. Differences in ways of knowing the patient were discussed and reviewed during report, but before this took place the admission narrative about a patient was recorded in the nursing records.

Recording the admission account

The admission narrative superseded the pre-admission account and was written in the nursing record. This was commonly referred to as the Kardex, and had an implicit sequential problem-solving design. It consisted of a pre-printed assessment sheet, a care plan and a free text continuation sheet. Additional patient information was recorded on observation charts that were kept by the patient's bed.

The assessment sheet had three sections – a patient identification section (name, age and next of kin), a medical information section (previous medical history, treatment, reason for admission and consultant) and a nursing assessment section. The nursing section was divided under Activities of Daily Living headings (e.g. mobility, dressing, hygiene) in which nurses recorded information, patient's remarks and comments about identified needs or problems.

Blank template care plans were available to produce a bespoke care plan. These had headings of identified needs, goals and corresponding action steps. Some pre-printed care plans had been introduced in an attempt to reduce the written work of the assessment, but these were not always adapted to the needs of the individual patient. In written and pre-printed care plans the associated action steps were not always recorded.

A free-text patient's progress report of care and treatment was written on a continuation sheet. As a contemporaneous record, these notes were written at least once per shift and sometimes more frequently, depending on what was happening to the patient. Progress reports were typically brief, except when the nurse thought that the patient was likely to complain. Differences did exist in the content of verbal and written narratives about the same patient (these will be discussed in Chapter 4). Once the assessment was completed and records written, the narrative was told to the next team of nurses commencing duty during the shift handover report.

Narrative development stage 2: Report

> *I always ask in report . . . you need to know what is happening to the patient.*

Shift handover report was the principal occasion when information about patients was told to other nursing staff. This involved a cyclical process of narrative giving, taking and discussion. It was then followed after report by narrative development by each nurse as they worked with patients. This cycle was repeated on every shift, every day and every week, and led to each nurse personally owning a patient narrative to the extent that they could claim to *'know the patient'*. Evening and morning reports had different lengths on account of the shorter 15-minute shift overlap at the start and end of the shift (morning, 7.45–8.00 a.m.; evening, 9.15–9.30 p.m.). A longer report, lasting up to an hour, took place during the lunchtime shift overlap (1.30–2.30 p.m.). All reports had a general format that was adapted according to how well those listening knew the patients.

The process of report

Nurses giving report referred to the Kardex and their own personal note sheet along with personal recollections of having cared for the patient. Nurses habitually began report by reading details from the Kardex: *'At report I tend to follow a set pattern from the Kardex.'* These included patient identification (*'name, age, date and reason for admission'*), recent care, treatment and changes in treatment. Each individual patient report ended with a verbal signal which indicated that the nurse was moving on to talk about a different patient. This was usually a rhetorical question, such as *'OK?'* or *'all right?'*. The first report given about a patient was typically formulaic and focused on tasks requiring completion and work in support of diagnosis or treatment.

The content of report

Nurses giving report were selective about the amount of narrative content that they provided, according to their expectations of what others should know about the patient. Nurses were asked if they knew the patients – *'eyes down, were you all on duty yesterday?'* – and if they replied *'we know him'*, the content of report was limited to patient identification information and remarks about changes to the patient's treatment or care: *'I always give name, age, diagnosis and then any changes and tests done.'* Nurses who claimed to 'know' their patients tended to focus on narrative change: *'I only tell what has changed after that.'*

Sometimes the narrative content was deliberately limited because experienced staff held the view that other nurses should make an effort to know each patient: *'I try to keep it to a minimum because you should know your own patients.'* This popular comment placed the emphasis on each individual nurse taking the initiative to check it and to seek information for themselves: *'A lot are like me and only give what I give. I like to get a full history and go and look it up myself.'*

The time available to give report also influenced how much information was given and how much discussion was permitted. The nurse giving report regulated it to accommodate open discussion or manage interjections. Sometimes these interjections were limited due to time pressure to *'move the report forward'*, or because the nurse was keen to get off duty on time: *'I've got to get off* [duty].*'* Occasionally interjections were simply ignored and the nurse continued to give report.

Nurses listening to report also had views on the level of information required, and report was the primary place where it was found. When returning after several days off duty, a nurse explained *'I haven't got time to look at what happened three weeks ago, so I ask at report. The information is important and I try to get as much as I can. It might have happened on a previous shift but might be relevant in the future.'* She went on to add that *'I always ask in report – they give a lot of irrelevant information, like who has had a bath . . . but you need to know what is happening to the patient.'* Later on she checked *'the notes for the results and tests and things like that'*.

Even when time was limited nurses sought specific information such as *'All observations, fluid balance, how they are doing medically, how they are feeling, e.g. low in mood, how the physiotherapist got on with them, the occupational therapist's input, and medical social worker referrals, the home circumstances, whether the family is involved and if there is anything they want doing.'* This highlights how the nurse collated a range of information with regard to nursing, care management and medical categories to develop their own narrative of the patient. Different reports had different functions. Short reports focused on continuing care and treatment plans, whereas long reports allowed more time for group discussion and narrative revision to take place. These will be examined next.

Narrative giving: short reports

Short reports were brief, lasting little more than a minute, and were given on the day-to-night and night-to-day shift handovers. They were pithy portrayals of how the patient was known, and included three categories of information (nursing, management and medical) and judgements representing information processing within and across narrative categories. Two examples are given below.

Day-to-night shift report

> *Mr Jones, 51, Parkinson's disease. In for PD medication review, stiff tremor on left side plus at rest with freezing episodes, nice man, general bath given, transferred plus two, diet and fluids taken OK. He was shattered post bath, hourly position change, likes cream – sacrum dry, transfers plus two, the physiotherapist gave him a rollator, but he's not steady or safe with two, the doctor said that he can be discharged when his wife is back. GP to start a drug treatment and then to readmit him for assessment to see if there is any improvement.*

Night-to-day shift report

> *Mr Armand, 21, a Muslim, diagnosis, symptoms.* [She questioned the diagnosis and then confirmed an original date of diagnosis in the nursing record as being March 1999.] *Dependent, past medical history, no allergies* [reading from the nursing record]. *On haloperidol, got an m.s.u. – nearly* [laughs]. *It is still needed. Was bad on Tuesday but OK last night.*

A summary of the different elements of these reports is given in Table 2.1. The narratives contain three information categories (nursing, management and medical) implying the use of a conceptual lens. Individual judgements associated with a particular category reveal how the patient is known as an individual as seen by the nurse as carer (*'shattered'*) and as an object of care by the nurse as care manager (*'dependent'*). A global judgement made across all three categories (*'nice man'*) represents how he is known overall as a person in relation to the healthcare team. References to investigations highlight information seeking in support of medical diagnostic decision making.

Although brief, and focusing on continuing care rather than opening up discussion for change, these reports did not refer to a written care plan or prescribe nursing care tasks to those listening to them. This implied that nurses were expected to 'take' the narrative and use it to decide for themselves the patient's care needs on that shift.

Table 2.1 A summary of the narrative information category content of short reports

Shift report	Narrative judgements	Narrative categories	Narrative information
Day to night	Patient known as: • Nice man	Nursing	• *General bath given, transferred plus two* • *Diet and fluids taken OK* • *He was shattered post bath* • *Hourly position change, likes cream – sacrum dry* • *Transfers plus two* • *The PT gave him a rollator but he's not steady or safe with two*
		Medical	• *Diagnosis* • *GP to start a drug treatment and then to readmit him for assessment to see if there is any improvement*
		Management	• *Name, age* • *In for PD (Parkinson's disease) medication review* • *The doctor said that he can be discharged when his wife is back*
Night to day	Patient known as: • Was bad on Tuesday but OK last night • Dependent	Nursing	• *Obtained an m.s.u.(urine specimen)*
		Medical	• *Diagnosis, symptoms* • *Past medical history* • *No allergies* • *On haloperidol*
		Management	• *Name, 21, a Muslim*

Narrative giving: long reports

Long reports were given at the lunchtime shift change and allowed time for discussion and narrative revision through a process of challenge, corroboration and validation. These contrasted with short reports, which often went unchallenged (or had any challenges limited) and were passively corroborated. Some long reports did pass without challenge, especially when the patient was 'known' by the nurses and the care and treatment plan had not altered. A typical sequence of narrative giving for a long report follows, and is summarised in Table 2.2.

> *Mr Vincent, 60, came in with chest pain and an intralateral MI* [heart attack], *TIAs* [transient ischaemic attacks – blackouts] *for the last 6 months, he had streptokinase* [an anti-blood-clotting treatment] *in A and E on the 21st. A quiet chappie, he spent the morning lying on his bed, not saying a lot, barely got an answer. Taking diet and fluids well, quite independent.*

This report follows a sequence of the nurse giving patient identification details (read from the Kardex) and narrative category information. Nursing category information included observations, the patient's mobility, communication and nutritional needs. Medical category information included a previous medical history ('*TIAs for the last 6 months*'), diagnosis ('*MI, TIAs*') and treatment ('*had streptokinase*'). Two judgements summarise how the patient is known. One is a global judgement about the patient's character in relation to the healthcare team ('*a quiet chappie*'), and the other is about his response to healthcare management needs ('*quite independent*'). As with short reports there was an absence of prescriptive instructions about the care to give, which again suggests that nurses were expected to identify the patient's needs and make their own decisions. The narrative being given was discussed during these reports.

Table 2.2 A summary of the sequence of a long report

Narrative-giving sequence		Narrative data	Narrative categories
Patient identification and management	Reading from a nursing record	*Name, 60, came in (date) with chest pain and an intralateral MI*	Management (of care)
		⇓	
Nursing category	Nursing practice focus	*He spent the morning lying on his bed, not saying a lot, barely got an answer, taking diet and fluids well*	Nursing
		⇓	
Medical category	Medical narrative; treatment plans	*TIAs for the last 6 months, he had streptokinase in A and E on the 21st*	Medicine
		⇓	
How the patient is known	Summary judgement	*A quiet chappie, quite independent*	Management (of care)

Discussing the narrative during long reports

These discussions involved challenge, corroboration and validation. Challenges were made to check information as it was given, as in the following conversation between two staff nurses:

> SN John (giving report): '*Mr Davies, 64, TB, meningitis, revision of shunt, no allergies, to contact physiotherapist and occupational therapist for continuing care form. She needs to do it.*' He verifies this by referring to the Kardex.
>
> SN Alex: Discussed details of the occupational therapist's involvement.
>
> SN John: Questioned whether the occupational therapist needed to be involved and continued with the report: '*full bed bath, 2-hourly care given, rested 06.45F. Feed on at 10.45, nil aspirate.*'
>
> SN Alex: '*Has he had feeds since 10.45?*'
>
> SN John: '*Yes – back on jevity plus* [a liquid food]. *He is awaiting private hospital, catheter, obs satisfactory.*'
>
> SN Alex: '*Is he opening his eyes?*'
>
> SN John: '*Yes, he is.*'

Discussion allowed other nurses to add information to the narrative being given and to corroborate or challenge what was heard. In Chapter 3, differences in narratives about patients are discussed to illustrate how report included challenge, corroboration and group validation. Discussion during long report giving supported the development of a group consensus on how the patient was known through contributions from different nurses.

During report, nurses also jotted down their own informal notes on scraps of paper. These were occasionally referred to in subsequent reports and during caregiving to check whether any outstanding tasks needed to be completed. The purpose and role of note sheets are examined further in Chapter 4.

So far an explanation of the narrative development cycle has included a pre-admission account, an admission narrative, record keeping and giving, and taking the narrative during report. The final part of the cycle is completed when nurses go to care for their patients.

Narrative development stage 3: Caregiving

> *From report, I make some notes and then go and look at the patient.*

After report nurses usually went directly to care for patients, generally without referring to nursing records. *'I go down the ward, get them up for breakfast, make sure they are comfy, get them washed, help with breakfast, get them ready for whatever they are going to do. I don't read the notes – I go and see the patients. I look at the patient and check what I think. I check how well they are, are they blue or not, if they are ready to get up or want to be left for a rest, or if they are wet they need seeing to straight away.'* Their interaction with patients provided an opportunity to check the narrative, add new information and develop personal ownership of it as they developed knowledge of the patient.

Several information sources could be drawn on to develop the narrative. Various staff members could be consulted to find out information, including nurses, doctors, relatives, physiotherapists, occupational therapists, dietitians, radiographers, porters and pharmacists: *'If I'm working with another qualified nurse I will discuss the care and what we need to do, it is a joint thing really, but if I'm just with untrained I will chat with other team members.'*

Information seeking also included narrative checking to detect change. For example, a patient's level of pain was checked by *'looking at the patient, his position in the bed and how he twists his body and groans when moved'*, and judgement of change was made in relation to the existing narrative. He was *'seen to be in pain by nursing staff, had spent an uncomfortable night and already had been given 10 mg stat of diamorphine in the past 24 hours'*. When adding to the narrative, some nurses saw the patient as a subject of care, and valued talking with them in addition to drawing upon other information sources: *'I talk to the patient, their family, do my own observations of their appearance and general health, also look in the medical case notes.'*

The narrative development cycle was completed through this third step of patient contact, information seeking and checking. New information was added and processed so that the latest development of the narrative could be told to nurses at the next report, as well as being used during the shift to identify the patient's current needs as the precursor to deciding on appropriate interventions.

Conclusion

Nurses' decision making has at its heart the creation and development of a narrative, which is an account of how the patient is known. The narrative originated through processing referral information into a pre-admission account or impression of the patient. This was subsequently revised following the patient's arrival on the ward through the nurse's involvement in seeking information directly from the patient. A nursing record includes an abstract of the narrative, and is referred to when giving the admission account to other nurses during report. The other nurses took report, listening to the narrative and often making their own informal notes on scraps of paper. After report nurses typically proceeded to care for their patients without reading the nursing record. As they cared for patients they checked the existing narrative and added new information, thus developing it. The nursing record was routinely updated towards the end of the shift. The revised narrative was told to nurses at the next shift handover report. The narrative development cycle continued from shift to shift and from day to day as a contemporaneous account of how the patient was known as they progressed along the trajectory of care. The whole purpose of the narrative development cycle was to know the patient and use this knowledge to identify the patient's needs and select interventions in relation to these. Knowing the patient in terms of three narrative categories (nursing, management and medical) was at the heart of decision making. Decision making is bound up with how patients are known, and the following chapter will examine some different ways of knowing patients.

Chapter summary box

- Narrative development and use are at the heart of real-world clinical decision making by the ward team.
- A patient is known by nurses through a narrative which is their account of them.
- A narrative has three categories of knowing, corresponding to the roles of the nurse as carer, care manager and medical assistant.
- A narrative begins when referral information is processed to form an impression of the patient. This is the pre-admission account.
- The admission narrative (account) is developed as the pre-admission account is checked and revised through direct observation and an interview discussion.
- The admission narrative is told to other nurses during report.
- During report, nurses listen to the narrative and make notes as part of the process of remembering it.
- Following report, nurses care for their patients and check the narrative to develop it by adding new information to produce a revised version.
- The revised narrative is told to nurses during the next report.
- A narrative development cycle involves giving and taking during report, checking and development during direct caregiving, and giving the developed narrative during the next shift report.
- The narrative is used in preference to the written record to identify the

> patient's needs, and forms the basis of nurses' real-world decision making.
> • The narrative develops as the patient moves along the care trajectory, which is the journey through the experience of healthcare.

Stop and think

This chapter has introduced the narrative of knowing the patient as being at the heart of decision making. The following questions ask you to consider the extent to which the narrative model helps to identify and explain aspects of your own clinical decision-making practice. The way in which you make decisions might differ, in which case the narrative model could be useful as a reference point from which you identify local differences and similarities.

Pre-admission

- How do you first hear about a patient being sent to your clinical area?
- What information do you receive?
- How do you make sense of it to categorise the type of patient and their needs?

Admission

- How is the admission process planned?
- Which documents are used and how does their use influence the type of questions and thus the information that you seek?
- To what extent do joint nurse–patient discussions constitute your admission assessment?
- What are the implications of conducting a largely one-way information-seeking interview with the patient?

Information sources

- Identify the range of information sources that you use during decision making and group them into different categories (e.g. verbal, written).
- Examine these categories and consider the quality of the information and its accessibility.
- What effect could restricted access to some information have on developing the narrative and subsequent decision making?
- Are there any information gatekeepers? If so, why do they have this role and what would be the effect on narrative development if their gatekeeper's role was to be removed?

- Could the information be made available in a different way (for example, electronically)?
- If so, would it support narrative development?

Information processing

- How do you process information and add meaning to it?
- How does information processing contribute to the way in which you develop knowledge of the patient?
- How does it direct your admission assessment interview?

Nursing roles

- What different nursing roles can you identify in your clinical setting?
- Do these add any additional lens facets to the conceptual lens outlined in this chapter?
- How do these roles revise your explanation of the phrase 'holistic knowledge of the patient'?

Report

- How do nurses giving report decide what to tell those listening to it?
- How is report conducted? Where does it take place and what is its content?
- How would altering the format and place of report shape narratives about patients?
- What formal and informal rules govern report and how do they shape narratives about patients?
- Analyse the information given in report and categorise it in relation to the roles that you have identified which nurses perform in your clinical area. Which roles are prominent in information giving at report and how does this shape how the patient is known?
- What assumptions are there about what every nurse should know about the patients they care for?
- Could report be altered in any way to promote knowing patients? If so, what would you recommend?

Recording narratives

- Do nurses compile their own personal informal note sheets during report?

- If so, when do they use them and what role do they play in knowing patients and organising nursing work?
- How are patients represented in the nursing record?
- How is nursing work represented in the nursing record?

(Records will be revisited in Chapter 4.)

Decisions

- What pre-admission decisions are made on the basis of the pre-admission account?
- What types of decision are made following the assessment interview and assessment narrative development?
- How are decisions represented in the patient's record?
- Which decisions, if any, are not written in the patient's record?
- Are there any factors that lead to decisions not being recorded?
- Could a change in practice alter what is recorded, and if so, what needs to be done?

Reference

1   Roper N, Logan WL and Tierney AJ (1980) *The Elements of Nursing.* Churchill Livingstone, Edinburgh.

Chapter 3

The narratives that nurses generate: ways of knowing the patient

Introduction • Narrative scope and depth • Information processing • Judgements within narrative categories • The ease of making judgements • Judgements across narrative categories • Ownership judgements • Ownership judgements and non-compliance with informal rules • Global judgements and non-compliance • Global judgements and the contribution of the healthcare team • Competing narratives • Conclusion • Stop and think

Introduction

Nurses know patients through the narratives that they construct about them. You might find that narratives about patients are a feature of your clinical practice and consider why it is easy to recall knowledge of some patients while less so for others. Part of the explanation for this lies in the scope and depth of a narrative. The scope refers to the inclusion of information in relation to the nurse's different roles, and the depth refers to the content of each narrative category. Nurses made judgements as they processed information to develop knowledge of the patient both within each narrative category and globally across all categories.

Narrative development included several nurses working in a complex clinical setting, and the potential existed to generate different versions of knowing the patient. This in turn led to questioning which narrative prevailed in clinical decision making. Given that there can be so many factors influencing real-world decision making, there has to be an explanation of how consistency and continuity of care is achieved. Two moderating influences shaped information processing and narrative development, namely the ward information hierarchy (individual peer review by more experienced staff) and group peer review (by the nursing team during report). There were times, for example, when different nurses in the same ward team had competing narratives with regard to whether a patient was lazy or ill. This had direct consequences for the decisions made about the patient.

Narrative scope and depth

In the previous chapter I explained how the conceptual lens could be used to describe how nurses' information seeking was shaped according to their roles within the ward. The information gathered was developed into corresponding narrative categories that the nurse interpreted to represent how the patient was known. Role influenced the scope of information seeking, while the extent of information seeking within each category determined the depth of information contained.

Narrative scope is a description of a nurse's use of one or more facets of the conceptual lens to seek information from or about the patient. It includes different combinations of the nursing, management and medical lenses. It follows that a limited-scope narrative will represent knowing the patient differently to a narrative that has a full scope. For example, a nurse and management lens combination supports knowing the patient as a person to be cared for coupled with overseeing their progression through their hospital stay. Such narratives are likely to include information and judgements about the patient's character, their stated requirements, and how they are responding to their own care and health problems. A medical and management lens combination, on the other hand, supports knowing the patient as a case to be managed, and can depict the patient as an object more than as an individual who might want to be an active participant in what happens to them.

Junior nurses were described as having limited-scope narratives: *'The junior will say in a report ''fine, eating and drinking'' and stay on a safe base. The experienced nurse will talk about the family details and contacts and have a lot more at their fingertips.'* This had a direct effect on recognising the need to make a decision: *'When results come in we will have a look at them and act on it – e.g. ring the doctor about a blood result and see if he will come up and prescribe some treatment such as blood. A junior wouldn't.'*

Narrative depth refers to the content of information generated in each narrative category. As nurses spent more time with the patient and developed their narratives, these categories contained a greater wealth of information. This contributed to their ability to remember the narrative to the extent of describing the patient as 'known'.

When taken together, narrative scope and depth referred to the quality of the narrative held in the mind of each nurse. It was revealed as nurses told their narratives during report and recorded aspects of it in the nursing record. Information loss in written records meant that the verbal narrative given in report could have a greater scope and depth and so became a more valuable source of finding out about the patient. This difference is dealt with in Chapter 4. Information was processed within and across the narrative categories and involved making a series of judgements. It was intrinsically linked to each nurse's knowledge and experience. This aspect will be revisited in Chapter 6 when explaining a trajectory between inexperienced, experienced and expert nurse decision makers.

Information processing

Information processing involved a series of judgements either within or across narrative categories. Judgements within narrative categories generated summary statements about the patient's health. Global judgements were made across narrative categories and included ownership, compliance with ward rules, non-compliance and judgements locating the patient in relation to the contribution of the healthcare team.

Judgements within narrative categories

Judgements made within narrative categories included comparisons between two states, such as observations of, or comments by, the patient. These types of judgement were statements of change or no change in relation to a particular aspect of information. When referring to health status this could be change as improvement, change as deterioration, or stability as a statement of no change.

In the following report, two judgements were made about the patient: *'Mr Jones, 59, acute sob* [shortness of breath] *exacerbation of COAD* [chronic obstructive airways disease], *history of hypertension; 100% better; IV discontinued; absolutely fine – doing own thing.'*

The first judgement of improvement change is *'100% better'*, in which the baseline reference is *'exacerbation'* of a respiratory problem. The second judgement implies an improvement, *'absolutely fine – doing own thing'*, suggesting independent activity, but does not include the baseline of 'not being fine' that was the health status when the patient was admitted to the ward.

Judgements of health deterioration included statements of *'he's going downhill'* and *'he's worse than yesterday'*. As with health improvement judgements, these were comparative and included concepts of movement (along an imagined health continuum), such as *'going'*, *'deteriorating'* and *'on a decline'*.

Judgements of health stability indicated that there was no change between reporting periods. Often during report a convalescing patient who was known by the team would be briefly identified along with a diagnostic label, and a judgement statement would be made about no change in his health and treatment or care programme (*'Mr Stanley, you all know him; MS, no change'*).

The ease of making judgements

Prolonged involvement in patient care facilitated information processing through accrual of knowledge about the patient: *'You meet them and see them and gauge how they are. You're able to just look and see how they are. You can soon know. You can judge quite quickly if you have been having someone for a long time.'* The process involved thinking through: *'You compare with your mental image to assess the change.'* One nurse gave the analogy of a mother–child relationship in which minor changes were detected even if the specific details were not consciously identified. There was a state of just 'knowing' that a change was occurring through comparison of current observations of the patient with the existing narrative about them. One part of knowing the patient included making global judgements across narrative categories.

Judgements across narrative categories

Global judgements were made across narrative categories and represented the patient both in relation to the healthcare team and in relation to the limits of the contribution made by the healthcare team. Judgements about the patient's relationship to the healthcare team included statements about ownership and compliance.

Ownership judgements

I'm taking him home for a garden gnome.

During a lunchtime report a nurse commented *'I'm taking him home for a garden gnome.'* The remark caused smirks but was not challenged. This represented a judgement about the patient as an object to be owned, which in turn implied an owner (the nurse). Although a gnome might be an object of affection or humour, this comment implied that an emotional distance existed between the patient and the nurse. There could be a reason for this, as it facilitated taking prescriptive care management decisions, such as where the nurse chose to place the patient in the ward. A staff nurse implied in her explanation of managing patients' activity how she had *'sat them in a day room until it was time to return them to their bedrooms'*. Referring in this way to patients rather than to individuals supports a process of objectification where the locus of control for decision making can move further into the nurses' domain. Information was interpreted to identify tasks to be completed, such as giving medication and bed bathing, in which the individual was cast as a passive object and as the focus of care tasks. Labelling the patient as an object (a gnome) moved this on a step further, and although it might have been intended in the context in which it was said as an expression of fondness for the patient, it nonetheless revealed far more about nurses approving particular characteristics of patients' behaviour. In this case one characteristic was compliance which lent itself to the role of nurse as manager/caregiver and the patient as object/recipient. Judgements that cast the patient as an object did influence practice to the extent of speaking at them or about them in their presence. For example, two staff nurses were checking on elderly patients in a four-bed bay early one morning. One nurse called to the other *'I need a bit of help getting him into bed. I fed him and he's still slipping down in his chair.'* Her colleague told the patient *'We'll put you in bed as the chair is not being any good for you'* and then said over the man's head to the other nurse, while holding him, *'He drinks quite well from a cup. I'll put him in a shirt – use one of our own.'* Throughout this episode the patient, an elderly man, was not included in their discussion or in the decisions that were being made about him.

Remarks about a patient's attempts to make autonomous choices also implied challenges to nurses' assumptions of ownership. An experienced staff nurse who reported *'He will eat and drink but only when he wants to, you know what I mean?'* implied a plan to get the patient to take food and drink as the nurse thought appropriate, which was countered by the patient's own choices.

Further challenges to ownership occurred in judgements linking the patient's behaviour to their mental state. The judgements in the statement *'He is barmy, a sandwich short of a picnic, he is like a ferret, in and out of everything'* liken the patient's inquisitive behaviour (*'in and out of everything'*) to that of an animal (*'like a ferret'*). Certainly the transition from a person to a non-person is evident here, and the supporting rationale is provided in a judgement of altered mental state (*'barmy'*).

Ownership judgements also located the patient in relation to nurses, especially when challenges to their decisions threatened their control over the decision process.

Labelling patients as compliant or 'good' referred to the lack of challenge made by the patient to the nursing staff. This was evident in judgements about patients who were *'all right because they don't give us a lot of trouble'*. Frustration with non-compliant patients was aired during reports. A staff nurse explained to her colleagues that *'in some way he is not an easy man to nurse – I feel like I have been banging my head against a brick wall'*.

This frustration was also influenced by the pressure that a nurse sensed if she was to be blamed for not carrying out a doctor's instruction. In the previous example the patient was expected to be a passive object in receipt of prescribed treatment, but whose non-compliance created a dilemma for the nurse. It was not the patient being proactive that was the threat, so much as the challenge to the status quo of hierarchical power which signified where the control of decision making lay. In this case the comment *'he* [the patient] *wants to have his say – there might be fireworks when he sees the doctor'* shows how the challenge rather than the content of communication threatened the status quo in the doctor–nurse–patient relationship. The nurse's anticipation of a reaction from the relatives also indicated how non-compliant patients threatened their ownership and control of decision making: *'He refused to put them* [pyjamas] *on. I don't know what his relatives will say.'*

Information processing within the narrative generated judgements about the patient that revealed a doctor–nurse–patient relationship and also how a nurse's role as caregiver, care manager and medical assistant could promote a view of the patient as a compliant object. The patient could be located in relation to nurses as an object to be owned and controlled. Patients were classified as 'OK' when this relational hierarchy was preserved.

The informal rules of this relational hierarchy were often only recognised when they had been broken. In the following incident the rule of being given permission to leave the ward was 'discovered' by a patient.

Ownership judgements and non-compliance with informal rules

> *I've only gone for a fag.*

Some patients were allowed, at a nurse's discretion, to leave the ward to go to the hospital shop, but most of them remained within the ward. The expectation that permission would be asked was not explicitly explained to patients or written on a notice anywhere. Apart from reasons of physical incapacity and the need to be regularly observed, patients remained on the ward for the convenience of medical staff. Doctors could visit the ward at any time to review a patient's treatment, and there was an expectation that the nurse would ensure that patients were available to be examined or interviewed. Given that there were several consultants attached to each ward, their teams of junior doctors did visit according to their own workload needs in each ward. These visits tended to involve a minimum of social chat with nurses and focused on completing medical tasks (reading test results, reviewing medical treatments and responding to nurses' requests). Patients who did not ask permission to leave the ward broke this informal rule and often were only made aware of it after they had broken it.

As Samantha, a ward sister, entered the hospital on her way to commence duty she noticed Shirley, one of her ward's patients, sitting in the entrance lobby. The NHS trust had a no smoking policy, so it was customary for several patients to be seen congregating around the hospital entrance to light their cigarettes. Shirley, a young woman, was sitting on a commode chair smoking a cigarette.

During the lunchtime report Sister Samantha explained to the nurses how she had asked Shirley what she was doing and was told *'I've only gone for a fag.'* Samantha recounted how Shirley was *'asked not to go again on a commode chair'*, at which the whole group of nurses listening erupted in laughter. The narrative during report majored on the humorous aspect of Shirley having used a mobile commode chair (as a seat) in public view. She had broken two informal rules, by inappropriately using ward equipment and leaving the ward without permission. The narrative about Shirley did not develop into one of problem patient and persistent rule breaker. The laughter validated this and an isolated single incident did not alter the narrative about Shirley into one of a non-compliant patient, nor was the incident associated with a deliberate challenge to the nurses' care management role.

Even patients who challenged the nurses and other staff were not necessarily regarded as non-compliant, and their behaviour was interpreted through the nursing lens as a response to health change. This occurred when Jane, a young woman, was admitted to the ward.

A few days after her admission Jane began to complain about the food that was being served on the ward. Samantha reflected on what the complaint was really about and interpreted it *'as a smokescreen really'*. She went on to explain her narrative about Jane and how she had *'lots of social problems, including three of her relatives who also were ill. One* [relative] *who had been in the intensive-care unit had since died, although this was before Jane had come to the ward.'* Jane's frustration was attributed to her physical inability to use her hands and *'overall she was looking increasingly tired'*. Judgements representing how she was known included *'frustrated'* and *'it was all getting to her'*.

One particular day, for a reason that was not given, Jane *'blew up'* at Samantha, stormed off the ward and was next heard of from staff in the visitors' dining room. A report was received that *'she had given a hard time to the kitchen staff and had thrown some food on the floor'*. Some patients in the ward had commented that Jane was *'out of order'*, and had been upset at having to witness the interaction. One of them had wanted to go home.

When Jane returned to the ward she denied having upset anyone, which resulted in some direct comments from other patients in her bay that she was a liar. Samantha mentioned how some patients had been *'sticking up for me, which was more than some of the other staff on the ward'*. The nursing team handled the conflict in different ways, suggesting that different interpretations of the narrative coexisted: *'One staff nurse did, the other male didn't and wouldn't get involved.'* A further challenge to the nurse's control of the patient within the ward occurred when Jane stated that she wanted to discharge herself. Samantha explained how *'I told her that I wouldn't advise it and that the doctors wouldn't take her back on very readily.'*

During her days off duty Samantha confided that she was worried: *'it's on your mind, isn't it?'* She revisited her narrative and mulled over what had been happening with Jane. During this time she spoke of feeling isolated from peer support: *'The senior sister was off, I carried a bleep, there it is – only 6 years post registration, and having been acting sister for 20 months. I didn't feel that there was anyone to talk to.'* When Samantha returned to work she *'left it . . . I didn't go and talk to her* [Jane], *she could have gone either way – blow up and here we go again, or an apology. It was difficult because I avoided her when I came on duty after my days off.'*

Her apprehension about possible further conflict made Samantha question the point of being a nurse: *'I feel that we do our best and then that's what you get. You feel that sometimes with all this why the bloody hell are you doing this, but I enjoy it really and so stick with it.'*

Samantha's decision was about what to do – whether to tackle Jane or not. This decision implied a global judgement of the patient in Samantha's narrative as a 'problem'. At some point Samantha checked her narrative: *'When I came back after my days off her attitude was different.'* She indicated that if it had not changed *'I would have had to formally sit down with her and discuss it, but as she had changed her attitude I decided to leave it.'*

The narrative was developed and this patient was no longer known by Samantha as a 'problem'. New information contributed to this change: *'Eventually she came and apologised and said she was out of order. I said fine, I'm just here to give you the best care I can. I feel that. I don't hold grudges, there was just a need to give her the care and then get her home. That's what she wanted, she wanted to get fit and go.'* Further narrative development depicted Jane as someone with improving health: *'I was on duty for two more weeks on nights and that was that, no more problems. She was so different after the steroid treatment. She got use back in her hands, looked refreshed and was like a different person.'*

Global judgements and non-compliance

> *Smart-arse sarcastic man.*

Non-compliance could be interpreted differently, and the patient's interaction with nurses did lead to global judgements being made about them in relation to nurses' care management role. Scottie became known for how he interacted with nurses beyond any considerations of knowing him in terms of his nursing care needs or medical treatment. As a result, the narrative about him developed from an initial judgement of *'all right'* to one of getting *'sick of it* [him]*'*. How this narrative development occurred is recounted below.

I was initially told about a 'problem' patient by Tom, a charge nurse. As I listened, I privately thought that he was giving a personal impression of the patient based on his own narrative rather than one shared by the whole team. However, during a subsequent report Scottie was described by a staff nurse as *'a smart-arse sarcastic man'*, who during his stay on the ward had initially been judged as *'all right'*, but soon became known as *'difficult'*. His continuing sarcasm towards the nursing staff had led to others in report confirming that they had *'got sick of it* [him]*'*, and they cited an episode of abusive verbal behaviour to confirm this. Moira, a staff nurse, updated the four staff nurses and two care assistants listening to report on what had happened over the previous two days when some of them had been off duty. The patient was no longer on the ward. Alan, a staff nurse, offered some background information about the patient:

> *We had a smart-arse sarcastic man. He played on it as well. At first it was all right, but we got sick of it. He also had MRSA. He was brought on to the ward and went down to theatre. When he got in the patient lift a few other staff also got in and made polite conversation. A medical records woman, just to make*

polite conversation, said 'You're in the best place.' He got angry, saying things like 'You're all right, you can walk, not like me', and he went off at her, swearing his head off. Everyone in the lift was embarrassed. I thought 'You childish little bastard – shut up.' When he was in theatre he was a bit warm and the nurse in theatre felt his head and remarked about it. He said sarcastically 'It's called a fever – don't you know that?'

Moira took up the story following his return to the ward: *'When he came back up to us post op. we got him transferred to a urology ward, giving the reason that it was because he needed urology care post op.'* Helen, a staff nurse, summed up the team's feeling of approval of this development: *'We were jumping up and down.'* A few days later, in private conversation, Tom validated the narrative and corroborated the decision that had been made: *'Later on, after a few days, he* [the patient] *met the staff nurse* [Alan] *off the ward and asked if he had been transferred because he was rude in the lift. The staff nurse said he had been.'*

What can be made of this narrative? The judgement across all narrative categories about the patient took a few days to develop, but did go through a transition from *'all right'* to being a problem (*'smart-arse'*). This was a result of compounding judgements shared by several staff over a few days during report. The corroborated narrative validated knowing the patient as a *'smart-arse'*. This validation was summarised in the phrase *'we got sick of it'*. Knowing the patient in this way impacted on the nurse's role as care manager and expectations of cooperation and compliance from the patient. Although the incident in the lift precipitated someone (whose identity was not known, but possibly it was Alan, who was in the lift at the time) to make a decision to seek Scottie's transfer to another ward, there was wider corroboration for this on the basis of Helen's narrative: *'We were jumping up and down.'* It suggests that the decision sought was right for the nursing team regardless of what might have been the appropriate place of care and treatment for the patient. An additional role of the nurse emerges here in that medical staff were implicated in colluding with this decision and authorised the transfer to another ward. The process whereby nurses influenced and challenged medical decisions through the nurse–doctor game is explored in Chapter 5.

Global judgements and the contribution of the healthcare team

It's tragic.

Another global judgement was the empathetic *'it's tragic'* type. An analysis of this in Table 3.1 shows how it was constructed across all three narrative categories as a broader interpretation of knowing the patient in relation to their hospitalisation and health change. This is evident in the following excerpt from a long report: *'Mr A Smith, 45, history – had on Tuesday a CT biopsy and frozen section, now diagnosed as astrocytoma. Wife to see doctor tomorrow, tragedy isn't it? She saw the doctor and is aware of it.'*

This global judgement was a statement about the patient's poor prognosis and an evaluation of the extent to which nursing and medical intervention could effect restorative health change. It influenced how nurses interpreted the patient

Table 3.1 A summary of a long report narrative showing how the patient was known as a tragic case*

	Global judgements (across narrative)	Narrative category judgements	Narrative categories	Narrative data
Lunchtime – long report	Whole nature of the narrative • *'Tragic'*	Character: • *'He is lovely'* Compliance: • *'An absolute gentleman'* Ownership: • *'I'm taking him home'*	Nursing	• *'Diet and fluids taken'* (nutrition) • *'Bowels opened small amount'* (elimination) • *'Catheter patent and draining'* (elimination) • *'Patient observations'* (monitoring) • *'He is an absolute gentleman'* (judgement) • *'I'm taking him home'* (ownership) • *'I'm taking him home for a garden gnome – he is lovely'* (judgement/ownership)
		Stability: • Judgement of instability	Medical	• *'Had on [date] CT biopsy and frozen section, now diagnosed as astrocytoma'* (investigations) • *'They have verified the diagnosis, discuss altering diagnoses?* (diagosis) *Treatment regimes, comments on size of pt for drug dose, note that CDs are due any investigations outstanding'* (treatment plan) • *'The nurse noted changes of type and doses of drugs'* (treatment plan) • *'She also compared the patient's current condition with previous observations (e.g. vomiting)'* (judgement)
			Management	• *'Name, 45, history – had on [date]'* (identification and chronology) • *'Wife to see doctor tomorrow'* (liaison) • *'She saw the doctor and is aware of it'* (liaison) • *'Transfer p.m. tomorrow'* (trajectory marker)

*In this table the data are grouped into narrative categories. Within-category judgements of knowing the patient are identified, and a global judgement is also identified across all three categories of knowing the patient.

and their actions. The term 'tragic' implies a sense of empathy with the patient's plight, and contrasts sharply with global judgements made about patients who were not cooperative or compliant.

Judgements within and across narrative categories represented information processing to construct how the patient was known. The process of report and the ward information hierarchy moderated and promoted an agreed way of knowing the patient. However, there were occasions when different narratives coexisted and this resulted in the patient being treated differently by different members of the same staff team.

Competing narratives

> *She's lazy . . . no, she's ill.*

A case occurred where a female patient was diagnosed as having a rare cerebral infection. Following a course of intravenous medication she was categorised as needing rehabilitation, and spent a few weeks on the ward convalescing. She tended to be lethargic. Most nurses on the ward had not nursed a patient with this type of infection before and were unfamiliar with typical patterns of post-infection recovery. Two competing judgements emerged about this patient. Some junior nurses focused on the need to progress with physical rehabilitation. The care plan recorded a broad goal of *'increase mobility'* under the Activities of Daily Living 'mobility' section, but lacked specific action step details and time-scales. The junior nurses had decided that the patient should comply with their interpretation of the plan of progressive exercise (e.g. sitting out of bed, supervised walking). However, the patient was frequently reluctant to get out of bed and even less inclined to attempt to walk. The junior nurses interpreted her lack of cooperation with their rehabilitation plans as due to her being lazy rather than incapable.

The senior nurses, in contrast, identified the underlying medical problem as the cause of the patient's response, and interpreted her state as lethargic rather than lazy. When they became aware, through a comment made by a concerned relative, that some junior staff appeared to be forcing the patient to mobilise against her wishes, they took action to regulate the agreed narrative. An information bulletin was retrieved from a clinical website that gave details about the infection and the typical experience of the patient. This was circulated to all staff, and was discussed at report and used to challenge the judgement that the patient was lazy. The peer-review role of senior staff established the global judgement of the patient as lethargic due to consequences of an infection, and discarded the competing view that the patient was lazy and posed a challenge to nurses' control of care management.

Conclusion

Narratives have both scope and depth. Scope refers to the categories included in the narrative, and depth refers to the narrative content. Information was processed by making judgements within and across narrative categories. Within-category judgements often referred to health change (an improvement or deterioration) or health stability. Across-category judgements represented the patient's relationship to the team (for example, as an object to be managed) and their relationship to the established hierarchy of decision control. Patients who challenged the status quo, sometimes by breaking informal rules, could become known as problems. This was not always the case, but when their behaviour developed a consistent pattern the narrative adapted to reflect this and the patient could be labelled as a problem. The nurses' decisions in those circumstances were directed towards managing the patient as a problem rather than focusing on the patient's problems. Thus a subtle shift occurred that tended to satisfy the nurses' needs as carers rather than the patient's care needs.

Narrative development was a team activity as well as the work of individual nurses. The team (through discussion during report) and individual nurses (through information hierarchy peer review) acted as a check and a balance on narrative development. The combined effect was to promote an agreed narrative. However, this did not always happen, and there were cases where patients were known differently and treated differently by different nurses within the same team. Narratives in nursing records were also different to their verbal counterparts told at report. These differences will be examined in the next chapter.

Chapter summary box

- The narrative has scope and depth.
- Narrative construction has individual and team involvement.
- Information processing involves judgement making either within narrative categories or globally across them.
- Global judgements include statements about the patient as compliant with informal rules and nurses' control over decision making.
- Global judgements include statements about the patient in relation to the contribution of the healthcare team.
- Different nurses can develop different narrative variants for the same patient.

Stop and think

This chapter has discussed the ways in which narrative information is processed through judgement making. These judgements contribute to making statements about how the patient is known. The following exercises ask you to consider your decision-making practice, particularly how you make sense of information processing, labelling patients and the effect that this has on the actions (decisions) that are taken.

Narrative scope and depth

- Reflect on your own decision making and identify cases where your narratives differ in scope. In what ways are the decisions different in narratives that differ in scope?

- Why are some narratives limited in scope?
- Are there any other developments in the narrative scope beyond the nursing, care management and medical lens described in this book? If so, what are they and how does this shape how the patient is known?

Different narratives about the same patient

- Identify cases where the same patient has had competing narratives. How did the difference arise and how was it resolved?
- To what extent are competing narratives evident in nurses' records?

Narratives and labelling the patient

- When processing information about patients, what types of judgement do you make?
- How do your information-processing judgements make statements about the patient in relation to yourself as a healthcare professional?
- To what extent do patients influence the global judgements that are made about them?
- Consider cases where global judgements have led to decisions being made about the patient that addressed nurses' needs to manage the patient rather than addressing the patient's needs. What can be learned from these cases? To what extent is it acceptable for the needs of the team to override the needs of the patient?

Chapter 4

Demonstrating narratives: differences between verbal and written narratives

Introduction • Why nurses write records • How nurses use records • The quality of written records and a need for change • How the patient is represented in a written narrative • Information loss between verbal and written narratives • The nurse's note sheet: an informal record • Conclusion • Stop and think

Introduction

Nurses make decisions through the creation and development of a narrative about the patient. These decisions should be recorded. There are many reasons why it is necessary to record decisions, including: professional obligation; so that the employing organisation can demonstrate that holistic, safe and effective care is being given; and fault trace when this does not occur, as part of governance and risk management. The patient also has a right to request access to their own records, and a court may subpoena nurses' records for use in legal proceedings. At the level of care delivery, these records should be used as a communication sheet by the whole team. It is interesting, therefore, to identify differences between the verbal and written narratives. The nature of these differences supports conclusions about the role of the written record in day-to-day clinical decision making. The implications of this necessitate revisiting the ways in which nurses work and the extent to which a document – be it paper or electronic – can capture what nurses do. Indeed, given that care can be given without recourse to written notes, it is necessary to recognise the value of the verbal narrative and to consider how that should be recorded.

I shall begin by examining nurses' accounts of why they wrote records, and move on to consider what they chose to write about their patients. An example of a care record will be compared with a corresponding verbal narrative to show how these differed and what implications this had for decision making.

Why nurses write records

Written records are necessary to satisfy organisational and professional requirements. The United Kingdom Central Council (UKCC)[1] and the Nursing and Midwifery Council (NMC)[2] require nurses to maintain contemporaneous records and to use them as a central feature of care delivery. This stance was at variance with the views of ward nurses, who did not support the notion of centrality, and described record keeping as *'documentation that we have got to do'* and *'a task to be done after giving care'*. Generally, nurses saw record keeping as something that *'had to be done'* for legal reasons, acknowledging the need to defend their practice against potential complaints: *'We might be dragged into court.'* The design of the record and the time available to complete it were cited as reasons why records were not central to caregiving. Peer pressure existed: *'I think they* [other staff] *spend too much time on Kardex'*, which suggested that writing was regarded as an administrative task rather than as work central to nursing care. Paradoxically, insufficient time was cited as a reason for not reading other records, even if they were thought to be relevant to decision making: *'If we had more time we would read the medical notes and find out more about the patient.'*

How nurses use records

Records were secondary to verbally communicated information, and were used for reference purposes: *'If I need to I will* [look at them], *but I get to know the patients and the discussion in report gives a picture before I go and care for them.'* Typical reference actions were to *'check something'* such as *'a lab report'* or *'to compare a written wound report with a current observation'*, and were part of judgement making about health change *'to see if it* [the patient] *had worsened or not'*. Nursing records were also used as a notepad or aide-memoire: *'It* [the record] *has a list of things to look for and check off.'* Nurses tended to refer to the record after spending time getting to know the patient: *'If I need to I will* [look at the nursing record], *but I get to know the patients and the discussion in report gives a picture before I go and care for them.'*

The question arises as to what else contributes to records having a low value in day-to-day care. The comment *'On here they* [records] *don't mean a lot . . . they get done . . . updated'* was linked to knowing the patient. One answer lies in the way that nurses described their work as based on thinking rather than on reading: *'I know the work off the top of my head.'* Ward sisters also concurred that a difference existed between real-world and theoretical practice (*'care is planned informally and the plans are written up retrospectively'*), thus lending support to the informal oral tradition of decision making.

Even in instances of apparently good record keeping, criticism was levelled at how accurately the patient was represented: *'Some* [wards] *are wonderful for care plans but* [these] *don't relate to how the patient actually is.'* Judgements about the quality of content, and thus about the implied fitness for purpose of records, strengthened existing views about their value in day-to-day caregiving.

The quality of written records and a need for change

Although notes were written contemporaneously with caregiving (a requirement of NMC professional guidance), there was some evidence that this did not equate with a real-time representation of the patient: *'If you look at these they are not kept up to date, and if you're honest I don't think that anyone does keep them up to date.'* Records were typically written retrospectively *'at the end of the shifts'*, two or three times each day. This relied on recall of events during the shift, as patient information is *'all kept in your head and then written up later away from the patient'*.

This resulted in omission of information because *'you don't get to write everything down at the time, and then when you are at home you remember it and the next day try to remember what you should have written'*.

Comments about the quality of records raised questions about where else nurses looked for information about what is happening with a patient. One source that was cited was a ward-round book. This was a notepad containing instructions given during ward rounds by medical staff, and it was *'better for report as it has the latest details from the round'*. It was described as:

> *a good source of finding up-to-date information as it has the latest notes on medical treatment, what doctors ordered on rounds, and can be used to quickly check back for investigations and results. In theory the staff should be able to go into the office to get information they need to answer queries. It is useful when relatives telephone the ward to ask when a consultant's round would be and what was said at the last ward round.*

This suggests that medical information was part of the narrative scope, and it hints at the dominance of the medical lens in shaping how the patient was known. Nurses needed to find out what was happening to the patient – shorthand for a nursing, medical and management summary – and the failure of records to demonstrate this was discussed by a specialist nurse. He described nursing records as *'sometimes okay for the social needs, but they are poor for real information. I find that they are vague and give continuous reports of ''had a good day, slept well and quiet afternoon'' but don't actually tell you what the shift was like for that patient.'* His remarks about needing to 'know' what is happening to a particular patient reveal an interpretation of the lived experience of the patient, a feature of the oral narrative. The volume of information within records, described by some as *'jumbled'*, did not always support narrative development: *'You . . . find yourself looking through piles and piles of paper in the medical and nursing notes. There are lots of pieces of paper and reports not filed in order, and it's very difficult to find what is going on with the patient. That is the problem – you can't go into the notes and find out quickly what is wrong.'*

The problem of poor-quality records (in terms of knowing the patient and what was wrong with them) led nurses to favour verbally communicated information: *'The notes don't tell you whether the patient is getting better, worse, or what. The notes are just a short comment, a change in treatment but without the discussion or reasons behind it. That's why the report is important to me, that's where I find out about what is going on. The care plans are so vague that two different people could give different care from the same care plan.'* It was more practicable to ask someone than to read through a patient's record.

Nursing records also included additional assessment sheets produced by non-nursing staff (e.g. a dietetics department nutritional assessment tool). These additions were regarded as *'irrelevant'*, *'vague'* and *'open to interpretation'*. Completion of these was also seen as a chore that was done grudgingly in order to avoid *'being picked up on if they didn't fill* [them] *out'*. Poor design, the time resource needed, poor quality and an apparent lack of fitness for purpose all contributed to these additional records having a secondary place to discussion in decision making.

This situation was freely acknowledged: *'We know that they should be central to care but are not.'* If this was to happen, change was needed that would have to alter nurses' existing practice of relying on verbal reports and their own note sheets. Nurses' informal practice was of little consequence in the face of legal, professional and organisational requirements, and it was recognised that a *'culture change was needed in nursing to get care plans to be used as a central document'.*

The time that nurses have available to write records, the quality of record system design and the real-time usefulness of other notebooks (e.g. a ward-round book), are all reasons why nursing records have a secondary role in real-world decision-making practice. Although nurses recognised their professional and organisational obligations to record their decision making, they prioritised attending to patient care over other considerations. They were aware of the legal implications of neglecting record keeping, but clearly the existing record system had deficiencies with regard to supporting clinical decision making. The need for change was recognised, even if the method of achieving change was unclear.

So far I have explored why records were written, how they were used and quality issues linked to questions about their fitness for purpose. I shall now examine the way in which the patient is represented in the nurses' record.

How the patient is represented in a written narrative

The assessment sheet

The written record consisted of an assessment sheet, a care plan and a free-text continuation sheet. The assessment sheet allowed different types of information to be recorded. It included information to identify the patient (name, age, address, NHS number, next of kin and preferred name), medical information (a brief medical history, current medication, diagnosis and medical reason for admission) and social information (such as type of home and dependants). This was all recorded on the first page. The next two pages were devoted to nursing care information based on an Activities of Daily Living model of nursing, and included sections for free text under headings such as diet, mobility, dressing and grooming. The fourth page contained some checklists for planning the patient's discharge from the ward.

The continuation sheet

The A4 free-text continuation sheet had three lined columns, the first for the date and time of entry, the second for the text and the third for the nurse's signature. The following narrative written on a continuation sheet is analysed to reveal the narrative categories and how these are interpreted to represent how the patient is known (*see* Table 4.1). This brief record, when analysed, demonstrated evidence of the different ways in which the nurse sought information about the patient using nursing, management and medical lenses (*see* Table 4.2).

In this narrative, the nursing, management and medical information about the patient located them on a care trajectory (type and route of admission). The medical information included a history ('*s.o.b.*' – *shortness of breath*), investigations, treatment and a marker indicating that the treatment process would not be initiated until the patient had been seen by a doctor ('*for review*'). The nursing information included observations of the patient's physical condition together

Table 4.1 Free-text entry in a continuation sheet

Date and time	Continuation record	Signature
10 March 1999, 10.20	*Emergency admission from coagulation clinic. Started with increasing s.o.b.* [shortness of breath], *chest pain and palpitations. On arrival on ward pain-free and palpitation settled, but continued to complain of shortness of breath. Very anxious on arrival. Simon states over the last few days he has been using his home oxygen more frequently and getting less relief from his nebuliser. ECG, bloods, O₂ at 2 litres.* *For review by medical doctor.*	S/Nurse Smith

with remarks about how they understood their health needs (*'Simon states . . .'*). The patient's remarks that were abstracted for inclusion in the record omitted any details about their perception of needs, or any reference to their participation in decision making. Information processing is evident in the judgement referring to the patient's health stability (*'palpitation settled'*).

This narrative focused on the patient's respiratory problem and represented them as a medical case being managed along a trajectory, denoted by the narrative marker *'for review by medical doctor'*. Two decisions were implicit in this record, the first about the nurse undertaking investigations to generate information for inclusion in medical diagnostic decision making (ECG [electrocardiograph], bloods), and the second about immediate treatment (oxygen administration).

Continuation sheets: sequential entries

Continuation-sheet entries could be brief, as in the example shown in Table 4.3 of a chronological sequence of entries made about a patient over a 24-hour period. An analysis shows how the patient was portrayed through nursing and medical narrative categories. Nursing information included remarks about hygiene, toileting and mobility, while medical information included cardiac monitoring, blood pressure recording and a report on a pacemaker function.

Information had been processed within these categories and included comparative judgements denoting health change – for example, *'dizzy'* (compared with not dizzy), and BP (blood pressure) *'shows significant difference.'* Others highlighted continuation of a particular health state – for example *'neurologically unchanged'*. The whole sequence lacked a global judgement about the patient, and recorded aspects of 'what is' but omitted references to care or treatment plans. A plan, whether formal or informal, is suggested in the monitoring activities reported.

The care plan

Care plans were written on blank template sheets (*see* Box 4.1). These were often kept at the foot of the patient's bed clipped to an observation board, or stored with the nursing record in the office. Regardless of where a care plan was kept, it was used infrequently and was only occasionally reviewed and updated. This did not

Table 4.2 Analytical summary of a free-text entry in a continuation sheet

Record entries (data)	How the data were labelled (data codes)	Conceptual lens category (data categories)	Interpretation of categories
Date/time, emergency admission from coagulation clinic	Type and route of admission	Management	The patient is represented as moving along a trajectory of care, and progression is currently paused until a medical officer has seen them. This implies that control of progression is, at this stage, dependent on the regulation of the medical officer
For review by medical doctor	Stage of narrative development	Management	
On arrival to coronary care, pain-free and palpitation settled	Nursing observation/judgement	Nursing	The nurse represented the patient's experience of ill health and their recent health trend. A judgement was used to mark the level of stability about one aspect of this trend (palpitations)
but continued to complain of s.o.b. (shortness of breath)	Nursing abstract of patient perspective	Nursing	
Simon states over the last few days he has been using his home oxygen more frequently and getting less relief from his nebuliser	Nursing abstract of patient perspective	Nursing	
Very anxious on arrival	Nursing observation	Nursing	
ECG, bloods	Medical investigations ordered	Medical	The nurse included three aspects of the medical narrative (medical history, investigation and treatment) that represented the patient as a case to be managed and an object of professional interest
O_2 at 2 litres	Medical treatment plan	Medical	
Started with increasing s.o.b., chest pain and palpitations	Medical history	Medical	

Table 4.3 Sequential continuation-sheet entries over a period of 24 hours

Date and time	Continuation record	Signature
12 March, 05.50	Neurologically unchanged, lying and standing BP shows significant difference. Mobile to toilet.	S/Nurse Smith (night shift)
12 March, 14.00	BM = 5.7 mmol at 12 md. Self-washed and showered with assistance. Dizzy this morning, shows no episodes observed or reported.	S/Nurse Adams (morning shift)
12 March, 14.50	Sitting BP 101/56, standing 90/50, pt starting to wobble slightly on standing for a long period. Measured for TED stockings.	S/Nurse Adams (morning shift)
12 March, 9 p.m.	Mobile with one. No c/o (complaint of) drop attacks.	S/Nurse Craig (evening shift)
13 March, 6 a.m.	Lying and standing BP recorded at 10 p. m., lying 90/56, standing 78/31. Doctors on call contacted and suggested cardiac monitoring. Visited pt and stated that monitor was showing that pacemaker was working. Up to toilet 3 a.m., felt dizzy, BP 88/49.	S/Nurse Smith (night shift)

mean that care was not planned or regularly reviewed. On the contrary, nurses developed their informal care plan incrementally through the narrative development process. Care plans had a problem-solving design that identified the patient's problems under an Activities of Daily Living category. Nursing interventions were stated together with a series of associated action steps.

Box 4.1 Blank template sheet for care plan

Name		Number	
	Activities of Daily Living category		Date/time
Problem			
Aim			
Action steps	1		
	2 etc.		

A limited number of pre-printed care plans were used, which addressed selected tasks, such as completion of the admission process. However, even though these had been an innovation aimed at reducing the amount of time spent writing records, many nurses preferred to write their own care plans:

We have pre-printed care plans, there are a number in the office. I prefer to write them myself – it makes you lazy, the pre-prints. We used to have computerised care plans, which I liked, but people didn't keep them up to date. If you look at these they are not kept up to date, and if you're honest I don't think that anyone does keep them up to date.

The staff nurse who made the above comment followed it with one that emphasised the oral tradition of care through discussions between staff: *'The care is discussed on a daily basis and you get to know your patients. You should be doing that anyway.'* When asked if care was planned informally, she replied *'Yes, things get sorted as they happen.'*

Even if care plans were used, they could be incomplete, notably omitting action steps, as illustrated in Box 4.2, which shows care plans with and without action steps. As was mentioned earlier, care was informally planned and delivered even if it was never fully recorded. On one occasion a patient had been admitted to a ward and received care for five days before a care plan was written.

Box 4.2 Care plans with and without action steps

Care plan with action steps

ADL category:	Maintain a safe environment
Problem:	Review medication
Aim/goal:	For tablet change to be effective
Action:	1 Administer medication as prescribed 2 Monitor effect 3 Offer support as necessary

ADL category:	Washing and dressing
Problem:	Hygiene
Aim/goal:	For high standard of cleanliness to be maintained
Action:	1 Offer assistance as required 2 General bath/shower as required 3 Oral hygiene 4 Change bed linen daily

Care plan without action steps

ADL category:	Maintain a safe environment
Problem:	Pt has reduced mobility
Aim/goal:	1 To regain his mobility to the best of his ability
Action:	(None recorded)

ADL category:	Breathing
Problem:	Pt has s.o.b.
Aim/goal:	1 To treat and relieve
Action:	(None recorded)

ADL = activities of daily living, s.o.b. = shortness of breath.

Information loss between verbal and written narratives

Nurses' support of the centrality of the narrative as the chief information source for decision making drew attention to information loss between verbal and written accounts of the patient. To illustrate this, Box 4.3 shows a comparison between a verbal narrative given during report and its written counterpart.

In this example both versions of the narrative included all three information categories (nursing, management and medical), but the verbal narrative consist-

Box 4.3 A comparison of written and verbal admission accounts

	Written narrative	Verbal narrative
Data	*'Patient admitted via A and E. Collapsed one day ago and now has right-sided numbness. Bloods (ticked), ECG (ticked), CXR, PEARL Venflon, BM 6.8 mmol. Baseline observations satisfactory, initial nursing observations satisfactory. Initial nursing assessment made, awaiting medical review.'* Signed SN Smith	The nurse explained having *'received a patient via A and E who came as a result of the pressure of the daughter. She had had a funny turn and collapsed, and was transferred on to Cherry Ward. No diagnosis as yet as she had been seen by the paramedics only. The patient was able to talk.'*

Accounts analysed by narrative category

Major categories	Subcategories	Subcategories
Management	Route of admission *'Patient admitted via A and E'*	Route of admission *Added* further data: *'who came as a result of the pressure of the daughter'*
Management	Management plan *'awaiting medical review'*	Management plan *Added* what was being awaited in the medical review (diagnosis) *'No diagnosis as yet'*
Medical	History *'Collapsed one day ago and now has right-sided numbness'* Bloods (ticked), ECG (ticked), CXR, PEARL Venflon	History *Added* details of the collapse *'She had had a funny turn and collapsed, and was transferred on to Cherry Ward'*
Nursing	Observations *'BM 6.8 mmol, baseline observations satisfactory, initial nursing observations satisfactory'*	Observations *Omitted* to state observations *Added* additional details about the physical assessment of the patient *'The patient was able to talk'*

ently added extra information. The additional information added context to how the patient was known, such as reasons why they were admitted (*'pressure of the daughter'*), the precursor to their collapse (*'funny turn'*) and a feature of their improving health (*'able to talk'*). In contrast, the written narrative included details of observations and investigation tasks that had been completed. Overall, the verbal narrative emphasised the patient who was ill, whereas the written account emphasised the illness associated with the patient.

The nurse's note sheet: an informal record

Nurses made notes at report on scraps of paper. These were kept in their pockets and were occasionally referred to during the shift. An analysis of these note sheets revealed a sequence of information recording that encompassed one or more of the three narrative information categories (nursing, management and medical). When these findings were triangulated with nurses' comments about their note taking, an explanation was formulated of the purpose of this informal record in narrative development. A typical note sheet written by a nurse during report about a patient is illustrated in Figure 4.1. Accompanying this is Table 4.4, which shows four particular features of the content (sequencing, annotations, colours and narrative categories), and Table 4.5, which shows the indicative content associated with each information category.

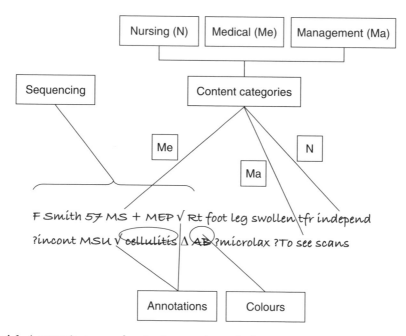

Figure 4.1 A nurse's personal note sheet written during report.

Note sheets like that shown in Figure 4.1 were written in blue or black ink and included annotations (circles, squares or underlining) which indicated the nurse's personal coding of tasks to be completed. Different colours were also used to denote priority tasks, such as red ink circles, and ticks were used to indicate task completion. For example, a confirmed diagnosis was marked with a tick as MS + MEP √. Mandy, a staff nurse, explained that '*I use two colours, blue for name, age, diagnosis, and red to highlight jobs to be done, like finding results.*' These were notes rather than longhand accounts, and included abbreviations such as Δ for diagnosis and AB for antibiotic. The information recorded matched the sequence given by the nurse in report, and included management, nursing care and medical information categories: '*It's things like name, age, what they came in with, past medical history.*'

Management information included patient identification ('*name, age, diagnosis*'), while nursing category information included Activities of Daily Living

Table 4.4 Four features of a nurse's personal note sheet written during report

Category	Content
Sequencing	Room, name, age, diagnosis, observations, ADL information
Content categories	Management – patient administration information
	Medical – diagnostic information/investigation information/ treatment plan information
	Nursing – nursing care (ADL) information
Annotations	Ticks – tasks completed
	Circles – tasks to undertake
	Underlining – priority of tasks to be done
	Box – priority of tasks to be done
Colours	Red – priority of tasks to be done
	Black – standard colour for recording notes

ADL = Activities of Daily Living.

Table 4.5 Indicative content of a note sheet associated with each narrative information category

Category	Indicative content
Medical	
Patient as diagnostic category	MS + MEP $\sqrt{}$ cellulitis (multiple sclerosis and cellulitis – a tissue inflammation)
Patient requiring treatment plan interventions	AB (antibiotics prescribed)
Management	
Patient as object in a liaison process	?To see scans (investigation reports to be brought to the doctor's attention)
Nursing	
Patient as recipient of nursing care tasks	?Incont ?Microlax (assessing whether the patient is incontinent and determining a possible nursing-initiated intervention to manage the incontinence)

issues, such as a mobility report that the patient could transfer independently (*'tfr independ'*) and a concern about their continence (*'?Incont'*). Medical category information included investigations such as specimen collection (*'MSU $\sqrt{}$'*), questioned whether or not the patient required an enema (*'?Microlax'*), and included a note about information to tell a doctor (*'?To see scans'*). The frequency of note taking was linked to the nurse's familiarity with the patient narrative: *'I only usually write stuff down if I have been off for a few days.'* More notes were made when patients were not known: *'When I come off holiday, like for 2 weeks, I have to take a bit more information and interrupt to remind them that I don't know the patient.'*

Note taking involved abstracting information from report because there was *'too much information to remember'*. It also helped to clarify what to ask: *'I sometimes ask more, depending on the type of report'* because *'some are not as factual as others.'* In doing so this called into question how relevant some reports were. Information was abstracted on the basis of personal relevancy: *'I write things down which seem relevant to me for that particular shift.'* This short-term focus, *'mainly about the specific tasks needed for that patient on that shift'*, was concerned with care management (*'what needs to be done'*).

The extent of note taking varied according to *'how much you know your patient'* and diminished to the point of being *'unnecessary after a few days of consecutive shifts'*. Once the narrative had been committed to memory, the note sheet as an aide-memoire was dispensed with. Malcolm, an experienced staff nurse, confirmed this: *'I get to know the patient and after a few days I have it in my mind what is happening with the patient.'* Likewise, Monica, a staff nurse, commented that knowing the patient was the overall aim of taking report, so she sought specific information during it:

> *I always ask in report, they give a lot of irrelevant information – like who has had a bath. You need to know what is happening to the patient. I look in the notes for the results and tests and things like that.* 'What do you write down at report?' *I only usually write stuff down if I have been off for a few days. Anything specifically I need to do I write down, usually a list of phone calls or other things that need doing straight away. I don't write diagnoses down unless I have been off, because you tend to get to know them, there is not that big a turnover on the ward.*

Once written, these notes were seldom referred to (*'once I have made a note of it I tend to remember it and don't need to look at it again'*), although some nurses did refer to them when giving report. The main purpose of writing notes was to remember the narrative so that decisions could be made: *'I pick up as much as I can, quickly, and filter it through my brain and plan something therapeutic for the patient.'* Knowing the patient and being able to give a narrative about them was valued by nurses, particularly experienced staff. However, those who could not do this courted disapproval from their peers.

This happened during a lunchtime report when a junior staff nurse did not know the patient that she was speaking about. She read from the Kardex old and possibly irrelevant information (*'Appendix operation in the 1960s'*). The other nurses in the room did not appear to be giving her their attention, and passed non-verbal signals (rolling their eyes) between themselves. Sensing this, she giggled, in apparent embarrassment, and asked the others questions to elicit additional information about the patient. No one responded to her.

The nurse's note sheet played a part in committing the narrative to memory and also served as a shorthand reference to prioritise and check on the completion of some tasks. Two systems were in operation with regard to decision making in the wards – formal and informal. The formal system involved compilation of a nursing record, whereas the informal system included ad hoc documents and the oral tradition of care. There was a difference between the two versions of accounts about a patient.

Conclusion

Differences exist between verbal narratives and their written counterparts. These differences modify the way in which the patient is represented. If the oral tradition of care is rendered invisible in nursing records, as indeed it is, additional information about the context of the patient is lost. It is this type of information that helps to explain the patient's experience of healthcare. Without such information the record can tend to portray the nurse's work as task orientated and dominated by a medical assistant role. Nurses' discussions about patients included more information about their experience of care and gave a broader representation of the nurse's role. This included nursing care (e.g. work with patients in physical and social realms), care management (e.g. liaison work, coordinating services and resolving conflicting plans) and medical assistant roles (e.g. gathering information to support medical decision making, and implementing and monitoring the progress of prescribed treatment). In addition, the peer review of narratives by experienced staff and the nursing team during report as part of the decision-making process is observable in practice, but is rarely detectable in the record. Differences between verbal and written narratives will continue to occur until the record system is central to decision making and is thus able to capture the process of decision making in a way that makes the record fit for its use and purpose. The existence of informal record systems in the form of nurses' note sheets and ward-round books highlights the fact that alternative systems are used as adjuncts to the oral tradition of care planning. Such records could be rendered redundant if there was a closer alignment between practice and the formal record system.

The implementation of electronic patient records represents a development in document design and is a tool for information management. However, it remains to be seen to what extent this development will impact on the merging of two parallel systems (informal and formal) into one at the heart of clinical decision making.

Narratives are at the heart of clinical decision making, and nurses use them to influence decisions outside the scope of their practice, namely medical decisions. How they do this will be examined in the next chapter.

Chapter summary box

- Nurses record their clinical decision making using a formal record-keeping system.
- This system is designed around a problem-solving approach to care, and incorporates a model of nursing.
- The existing record-keeping system does not capture the extent of information that is contained in a verbal narrative.
- The existing record-keeping system is not central to nurses' clinical decision making.
- Nurses use informal records (e.g. personal note sheets and ward-round books).
- Information is lost between verbal narratives and their written counter-parts.

- The verbal narrative adds context to information about the patient.

Stop and think

This chapter has drawn attention to the differences between the formal and informal representations of the patient in decision making. All clinical care settings that involve a team of staff will include multiple discussions about care, whether on a one-to-one basis or in a scheduled team forum. It is likely that in your clinical area more is spoken about care than is actually written down about it. The following questions are intended to prompt further exploration of what is lost between verbal and written accounts of your patients.

Formal records

- What formal record-keeping system do you use?
- Which models, if any, are incorporated into this record?
- How does the design of the record shape the way in which the patient is represented?
- To what extent does the record capture team contributions to decision making?
- How often is the record used during a shift?
- Should it be used more frequently, and if so, what would promote such use?

Informal records

- Do informal records exist in the clinical area?
- If informal records exist, what are they and who compiles them?
- How are informal records used?
- When are they discarded?
- If they are discarded, what is lost from inclusion in the formal record system?

Difference between written and verbal records

- Compare a written account of a patient from your formal record system with the verbal account given at report. In what ways are these similar and different?
- If there is a difference, how does it shape different representations of the patient?
- What impact does acting on different representations of the patient have on decision making?

References

1 United Kingdom Central Council (UKCC) (1998) *Guidelines for Professional Practice.* UKCC, London.
2 Nursing and Midwifery Council (NMC) (2002) *Guidelines for Records and Record Keeping.* NMC, London.

Chapter 5

The games nurses play: making narratives known to doctors

Introduction • Nurses, doctors and the context of clinical decision making • Different types of relationship between nurses and doctors • Improving nurse–doctor relationships • Non-confrontational tactics that are used to make narratives known • Confrontational tactics that are used to make narratives known • The historical legacy of resistance to recognising nurses' ways of knowing patients • Conclusion • Stop and think

Introduction

Knowing the patient is at the heart of an oral tradition of decision making in which the narrative is used to identify needs and match them to intervention options. Nurses' narratives are not the only way of knowing the patient, and other healthcare staff, notably doctors, can hold different views about the patient's needs with regard to care management and treatment. Nurses recognised this difference and used their own narratives to challenge doctors and influence their decision making. In this chapter the nurse–doctor relationship will be described together with the communication tactics that nurses used to make their narratives known to doctors.

Nurses, doctors and the context of clinical decision making

In ward settings tension existed concerning who owned and controlled the environment of care and the patient within it. Nurses claimed ownership of the ward on account of their continuous presence: *'The nurses are here all the time, 24 hours a day.'* Nurses have had responsibility for managing the environment of care since Nightingale's day through management of the patient in the sick-room (ward) to allow the laws of health and nature to act on them. Doctors had the role of intervention in the health and healing process. These responsibilities translated into contemporary nursing practice as a care management role with responsibilities for regulating a safe clinical environment through the oversight of health and safety arrangements, such as the ordering, maintenance and safe use of clinical equipment and the storage and disposal of hazardous substances and clinical waste. Nurses also coordinated the contributions of other staff who visited or worked in the ward. The ward manager was the hub of this process.

Doctors frequently assumed control of care and treatment when they were in the wards, and by implication challenged the scope of nurses' efforts to manage care. This has been recognised elsewhere. For example, Gair and Hartery[1] commented on how doctors saw the patient in the ward as their territory due to their legal accountability for patient care. Such challenges to nurses' claims of ownership were typified by remarks about doctors *'coming on as if they own the place'*, and provoked a response to reassert territorial control: *'The staff are good at dealing with bombastic doctors.'* Part of asserting this control included supervising or policing activity within the ward. For example, one sister worked around the office close to the ward entrance and monitored who visited the ward as well as the work that was going on within it. When junior doctors visited, she exerted her control by directing them to undertake tasks written by nurses in a communication notebook (such as inserting intravenous lines, collecting blood specimens and writing prescriptions). The clearest reversal of nurses' control of the ward environment occurred during consultant-led ward rounds, in which nurses were expected to ensure that patients and their records were present to be reviewed by the medical staff, and junior nurses had to keep away so as not to interrupt the round. It was in the context of nurse–doctor relationships that a particular communication game existed. Both groups had a stake in managing patients' care and treatment. Nurses assumed ownership of the ward and work within it. Doctors drew on their positional power within the organisation, and their claim of legal responsibilities towards the patient as a 'medical case', to assume a decision authority that directly affected the work of others in the ward. The nurse–doctor relationship was integral to shaping decisions made about the patient and about care management. So what was the relationship between nurses and doctors?

Different types of relationship between nurses and doctors

The nurse–doctor relationship varied from good to poor, with some doctors being regarded as *'likeable'* because they acknowledged nurses' views. Some doctors were described positively (*'he seems to listen'*), while others were referred to as *'horrible'*, *'aloof'* and *'rude'* because they *'didn't generally talk to nurses'* or patients. Poor relationships were attributed to the lack of interpersonal skills of doctors, not nurses, and were associated with a perception of how the doctor 'saw' the patient. This was principally from a medical case management perspective. Poor relationships were grounded in judgements about how doctors dealt with others, including an *'inhuman . . . bedside manner'* that was *'prescriptive'* towards the patient and *'dictatorial'*, *'arrogant'*, *'angry'*, *'disapproving'* and *'moody'* towards nurses. Senior doctors were implicated in influencing junior doctors' attitudes towards nurses: *'Some will only take notice when the consultant listens to you on a round, then they start to give you a bit of respect.'*

Nurses held a range of views about the doctor–nurse relationship. Junior staff were described as being *'a little in awe of doctors'* and timid in their presence. Some were *'uneasy'* when certain doctors were on the ward, and tried *'to keep on the right side of him'*. Circumspect timidity was compounded by previous experience of making unsuccessful complaints about doctors' behaviour: *'If we complain they* [doctors] *go to management; management always assume they are right.'* The organisational power of doctors was alluded to in comments made about the indirect pressure that they could bring to bear on nurses: *'They say* [to the hospital managers] *things like "I'm leaving if you don't do something about the attitude of staff."'* This could result in admonitions (*'you end up getting told off'*) or being sent formal letters: *'Consultants have occasionally sent letters criticising staff for reacting to doctors. We replied back that they come with the attitude that they expect a nurse to be at their side. We don't ignore them but go with them* [to see patients] *when we can.'* Experienced staff took a more confident stance, describing doctors *'not as some god, but here to do a job'*, and challenged the hierarchical doctor–nurse relationship: *'I speak to them like I always do.'*

Some junior doctors did seek nurses' views and asked for their advice about patient treatment (for example, *'what do you do here?'* and *'what do you think?'*). Nurses also regarded doctors' agreement with their comments as a form of *'peer review'* or validation of their narrative. This gave them *'confidence to approach doctors'*, particularly when acting as advocates *'for the patient'*, whether this concerned observance of hospital *'policy'* or presenting a *'challenge from the team* [nurses]'. Advocacy could be dismissed when it was seen as a challenge to medical decision making: *'It depends on the consultant. With old-fashioned doctors we make no suggestions as we know damn well that they will do the opposite to what we suggest.'* Other doctors did listen to nurses, even though there is implied decision authority in the reference to *'taking no messing'*: *'With others we can discuss the patient with them and make suggestions. Dr Marham we have known for a long time, he came through here as a senior reg., but he is strong and takes no messing.'*

Some consultants supported the sisters' role at the top of the ward information hierarchy and preferred only to speak with them. This gave rise to problems, as it was *'difficult when a lot of doctors come together'* and then did not want a staff nurse to accompany them on a ward round: *'You will get that with a consultant, they want a navy blue dress – even the younger consultants. Some are not as bad and will do a round with a staff nurse, but you can see that they want the sister on the round.'*

One aspect of doctors' attitudes towards nurses lay in their expectations of nurses' work and the information that could be given to support medical decision making. Nurses were expected to know their patients, specifically with regard to social care issues rather than medical details: *'They* [doctors] *expect you to know the patient and you try to give the information needed but don't get too involved in the rest of it. The social circumstances you need to know, and it is very embarrassing if you don't know it.'*

Some nurses recognised limitations in their ability to provide this information: *'It's a pain really . . . as doctor expects you to know more about the specific patient than you* [actually] *do.'* Sometimes they tried to deflect doctors' questions to hide their lack of knowledge by claiming that they *'had only just come on* [to the ward]'. Others questioned doctors' professional self-interest and their limited view of nurses' work: *'The doctors . . . come on and want the sister to go and attend to just what they want and don't seem to realise that she has staff as well as 28 patients to manage.'* Their approach towards nurses could be prescriptive and lack awareness of their wider role in the ward: *'A doctor came on to the ward complaining about a lack of equipment and gave the nurse an order. He said "just get it" and didn't want to listen to excuses. He thinks nurses are always having breaks and sitting down, but they don't see the whole picture* [of nurses' work].'

However, although nurses valued their own work, some acknowledged that its vague, 'airy-fairy' nature contributed to its invisibility: '*When we have a dependent ward it is busy with patient care. We see that as our nursing priority and are taken up with washing, dressing and feeding of patients. This is the important role of the nurse. That can take all morning and the doctors don't seem to appreciate it.*' Steps were taken to improve poor relationships, although these were not always successful.

Improving nurse–doctor relationships

Sister Julie explained how a doctor avoided discussing the problem of fractious relationships on the ward, stating that '*he didn't want a relationship with a member of staff*', but others were open to discussion: '*We can discuss the patient and make suggestions.*' Nurses also wanted good relationships to satisfy their own information needs: '*There is only so much info the nurse can give because the doctor doesn't always give the full picture and so you will really have to talk to him.*' Nurses could not rely on doctors always to tell them medical information about patients, and so resorted to reading the medical notes: '*I was looking in a set of medical notes to see the updated care of patients and discovered that a discharge had been planned without telling the nursing staff. Good of them to tell us* [said sarcastically].' There were occasions when doctors held private discussions in the ward office and only passed on brief instructions to the nurse in charge, without including a rationale. On other occasions they would make a note in the medical record and omit to inform the nurses. Neither act was satisfactory, as nurses needed to coordinate the management of the patient and make this meaningful in their discussions with them. Often they acted as an interpreter for the doctor, not from English into a foreign language, but from technical language to one that could be understood by patients. For nurses, knowing why the medical staff had made a particular decision was as important as knowing what decision they had made. Communication with doctors was vital to understanding the medical perspective and to making the nurse's narrative known so that they could act as a patient advocate.

Whenever nurses thought that medical decisions were not in the patient's best interest, they played a communication game to make their narratives known. This is called the nurse–doctor game. The goal of the game was to shape decision making, the focus was knowing the patient, the players were doctors and nurses, and the moves were communication tactics. The specific moves in this game included non-confrontational and confrontational tactics, such as making indirect comments, flirting, reasoning, refusal, going to more senior doctors and sanctioning a change in the locus of decision control.

Non-confrontational tactics that are used to make narratives known

Being 'unhappy'

Nurses indirectly challenged medical decisions by using non-specific phrases about the patient (not the doctor), such as '*not being happy*' or '*I'm concerned*'. This was non-confrontational as it was the nurse's statement of her own perception about a situation, rather than a direct reference to anything in which the doctor was implicated, as if the nurse was letting the doctor eavesdrop on her own private musings. However, it did signal an invitation for the doctor to discuss this concern further.

Flirting

Some female staff attempted to influence medical decisions by flirting with and flattering doctors. This was a deliberate ploy that went beyond normal social niceties such as including a doctor in a staff tea break on the ward (doctors never had lunch or took tea breaks with nurses in the staff canteen). They made doctors drinks, deliberately sat next to them, engaged in social rather than clinical conversation, and used their body language as a precursor to stating what they required. Sister Julie demonstrated this, after telling me that she wanted a doctor to change his decision. She flirted (by maintaining prolonged eye contact and making her breast profile visible to a doctor) and introduced in conversation the need to revise a patient's treatment plan. The doctor considered the nursing information provided and subsequently revised the treatment plan. If a junior doctor tried to flirt with nurses they were rebuffed and their actions led them to being privately described as a *'creep'*. This highlighted a difference in interpretation of the use of this communication tactic. Flirting was used on some occasions, but the norm was to discuss concerns by reasoning why a decision needed to be challenged.

Reasoning: improving care and saving lives

Reasoning was described as *'setting your stall out'* and was frequently used to influence medical decisions. Tom, a charge nurse, explained how he had successfully argued for the postponement of a planned operation for a patient who was due to have a percutaneous endoscopic gastrostomy (PEG) (a feeding tube inserted through the abdominal wall). He had judged that the patient was unfit to undergo the procedure (this was his global judgement about the patient within his narrative): *'The doctor was wanting to PEG a patient and I said ''not now, as I think that you would lose him''.'* Tom went on to add how he reasoned with *'Dr Smith that I needed three days to nasogastric feed the patient, build him up and then take him down for a PEG next week'*. Tom's view that without this delay the patient might die was accepted, and Dr Smith replied *'right, we will do that'*, with Tom adding, *'That's when they respect and listen to your judgement.'* Other nurses concurred with the use of reasoning: *'On a ward round, if you tell the consultant about a wound, you need to set your stall out and give reasons for what you did, not just a statement like I think that that will be best, e.g. this has a wick with an absorbent aquacell (dressing) and permeable pad on the top.'* Reasoning was not always listened to, so nurses might resort to confrontation to get the attention of the doctor so that they would listen to their narratives.

Confrontational tactics that are used to make narratives known

Direct refusal

Refusal of a medical instruction was a high-risk strategy that was likely to bring the nurse into sharp conflict with doctors, but did sometimes result in the nurse's narrative prevailing to alter the care management plan. Alan, a staff nurse, described a typical instance of this:

> A patient had diarrhoea and we don't start a treatment until we know what the causative organism is. The doctor wanted to prescribe loperamide. He was told that it was OK if he wanted to prescribe it but it wouldn't be given unless we knew the cause of the diarrhoea. You see if it was infectious diarrhoea and you give a drug to slow down the bowel, you can cause other problems such as toxic megacolon and the patient can become really ill, making things worse.

This direct refusal of a medical instruction along with a supporting rationale was likely to promote confrontation. It did not always deflect some doctors from insisting on their prescribed plan for the patient, so nurses exercised the option of ignoring the medical instruction and appealing for support from a higher-grade doctor. This in effect entailed using one of the same tactics mentioned earlier for which they had criticised doctors, namely being dismissive of their views. However, resorting to confrontational tactics implied the failure of trying to reason with doctors.

Going to more senior doctors

Referral to a more senior doctor was not readily undertaken. Persistent reasoning was often employed to make their narratives known, variously described as 'telling', 'reasoning', 'tell and tell again' and 'badgering' doctors. The threat of 'going to a senior doctor' was sometimes successfully used to pressurise a junior doctor to alter a medical decision. If they did not make the decision that the nurse thought necessary, a more senior doctor was contacted:

> We have just got a change of house officers and they are scared of their own shadow at the moment. They haven't got to know us and to trust our judgement yet. In that case I would go and bleep the SHO, who has been here a little longer and has a little more consideration behind their decisions. In this case she said that we could change the drug and she would come and write it up. She bleeped a house officer and sent him up to do it. That's why he questioned what the cancer nurse said but went along with it in the end.

This type of challenge could create tension between medical staff, and to avoid this situation developing, some junior doctors sometimes complied with the nurses' requests, especially when these focused on administration issues such as completing pharmacy prescriptions: *'I have had a run-in with a couple of them and have to go above them to the SHOs to get some drugs written up.'* The overriding consideration in making the narrative known to challenge medical decisions was the nurse's focus on the patient and their needs:

> *I will* [challenge the doctor] *on anything, that's me, junior staff will not have the confidence. I tell them that if they are not happy* [with some patient care] *then to tell the doctor, even to the point that I would ring the consultant if I was not happy. A couple of the juniors might not.*

Mary, a sister, went on to state her priority when dealing with these concerns: *'Ultimately the responsibility is nursing the patient and that's the point, not pleasing a doctor.'* Narrative-based decision making is all about patient-centred care – knowing the patient. The narrative could favour an emphasis on any one of the three categories of knowing the patient (nursing, management and medical), but it was the nurse primarily acting as an advocate and adopting a holistic view that encompassed a full-scope narrative which spurred on the challenge of medical decision making.

Although the doctor–nurse game existed, several factors shaped whether it was actively played. These included the nurse's confidence in the scope of their role, particularly their ownership of care management, their confidence in knowing the patient and their awareness of how different medical staff treated nurses. Whenever the game was played, control of patient management within the clinical territory was a foreground issue between nurses and doctors. There were occasions when doctors relinquished control of the patient. This was when the patient moved towards discharge from the ward.

Sanctioning the transfer of the locus of control from medical to nurse decision making

Once the medical staff had evaluated that the treatment plan had achieved particular goals, and there was no further need for the patient to be on the ward, they decided that the patient could be discharged. This suggested that the doctor had a veto on control of the patient along the care trajectory. Sometimes, when doctors made this decision and announced it to the nursing staff, it was immediately challenged:

> *A doctor will say they can go home and I will say 'Slow down, we have to get things sorted.' The doctors here do look at the whole and ask 'Sister, what are the social circumstances of this patient?' The nurses are good here for advocating what the patient wants; things are discussed with the patient to see if there can be a compromise if they don't want the care.*

At this point, nurses played the major role in overseeing the final progression of the patient to the end of the care trajectory and discharge from the ward. This included taking responsibility for a range of administrative and liaison tasks, and ensuring that there was appropriate referral to post-discharge support services. Although this represented nurses having control over part of the trajectory, it appeared to be at the sanction of doctors, which implied that this control could be transferred back to medical staff if the patient's medical condition altered and necessitated further medical intervention.

The historical legacy of resistance to recognising nurses' ways of knowing patients

Historically, challenges to medical decision making have met with resistance from the medical profession. The articulation of nurses' narratives and new roles with enhanced decision authority present challenges to the prevailing medically led ways of knowing the patient. This specifically probes the boundaries that preserve power, decision authority and interpersonal relationships within wards. It is not surprising, therefore, that a challenge to the status quo which preserves medical control over management and treatment of the patient along the trajectory of care meets with resistance from doctors. One example of this resistance is doctors' questioning of the direction of professional nursing practice, as noted by Maslin-Prothero and Masterson[2] in their comments on Short's headline in the *British Medical Journal*, 'Has nursing lost its way?',[3] which advocated a return to the 'old' nursing values. Maslin-Prothero and Masterson[2] made the point that it was unlikely that the work of medicine and doctors would be discussed in such a way in a nursing journal.

Resistance and the communication tactics used by nurses have been recognised elsewhere, particularly in Stein's '*doctor–nurse game*'[4] as a feature of medical staff hegemony in the clinical setting. Although Hofling and colleagues[5] wrote about it first, Stein[4] is attributed with labelling the relationship as a game. Its origin is in the '*essentially patriarchal*' doctor–nurse relationship[6] in which nurses had traditionally conformed to a gendered family role as a female carer, and it is characterised by a dominant–subservient male–female relationship.[7] The main rule of the game, according to Stein,[4] was that open disagreement between the players must be avoided: '*The nurse can communicate her recommendations without appearing to be making a recommendation statement. The physician, in requesting a recommendation from a nurse, must do so without appearing to be asking for it.*'

A later review of the doctor–nurse game by Stein *et al.*[8] concluded that nurses had unilaterally decided to stop playing it. Nurses, these authors claimed, were now hostile, stubborn rebels, and associated this with becoming autonomous healthcare professionals. In a similar way, Sweet and Norman[6] confirmed that although previously this game had been played '*almost without exception*', it was now rarely observed in hospital settings. This was attributed to broader changes in the improved status of women in society. Findings from the study on which this book is based suggest otherwise, principally indicating that nurses can play the 'stubborn' role but are also quite capable of adopting tactics or game playing to ensure that doctors hear their narratives, in order to influence medical decision making. These tactics were often used when vying for control of the patient's progress along the trajectory of care, and such 'turf wars' are likely to continue so long as there are differences in decision authority that favour doctors' ultimate sanction over nurses' decisions. Some of these differences are between nurses' and doctors' views of their roles in the ward. According to Snelgrove and Hughes,[9] doctors viewed themselves as the key figures in the management of treatment, so the decisions that needed to be made were essentially medical ones based on medical knowledge.

Similar comments to those discussed earlier in this chapter about doctors' attitudes towards nurses have also been reported elsewhere – for example, in the description by Adamson, Kenny and Wilson-Barnett[10] of doctors as *'authoritative, powerful, assertive, prestigious, autonomous and complacent'*. Castledine,[11] a nurse, attributed this *'arrogance'* to the way in which doctors see the nurses' role and their ignorance of what nurses are achieving. To be sidetracked into a medical assistant role was a move away from the *'real issues'* of professional role development. The recently coined term 'maxi nurse' further emphasises the development of nursing rather than a transition into medicine as a 'little doctor'. A lack of understanding of the role of nurses highlights the invisibility of their work to doctors. Nurses as advocates can provide a safeguard that actually protects the patient from decisions which could cause them more harm than good. Nurses' contributions have historically been selectively silenced.

Chiarella's analysis of Australian case law between 1904 and 1999[12] reported how nurses' voices and experiences were excluded to the extent that they were historically portrayed as little more than extensions of doctors. Furthermore, their actions were only given weight when the doctors said so. This represents successful medical hegemony, and the review by May and Fleming[13] of socio-logical accounts of interprofessional relationships concluded that nurses are subordinate to doctors. They went on to discuss how nursing is more concerned to construct difference than *'to compete on the same terms, for the same turf'*. The construction of difference, they claimed, had been given insufficient priority in sociological accounts. A departure from a purely medical model way of knowing the patient (that supported the generation of medical lens knowledge) was needed, which involved examining different ways of constructing the patient, not from distinctions arising from organisationally constituted boundaries, but through professional discourses. The doctor–nurse game represents the interface of this discourse at ward level, involving short-term interaction and game playing within the status quo of existing roles and decision authority. A wider discussion of reconfiguring the roles of clinicians in health service delivery is the place where more enduring change is likely to occur. With a latent professional tribalism as the subtext to this debate, some have accused nurses of adopting a strategy of closing themselves off from biomedicine to represent their work in terms of holism.[13] This was not found to be the case in the study that underlies this book, as nurses straddled the divide between themselves and doctors, standing on the common ground of patient management, which might be taken to mean the common *'turf'*[13] that was referred to earlier.

Conclusion

It is one thing for nurses to know their patients and make care decisions on the basis of the narrative. It is another for them to use their narratives to influence medical decision making. The context of ward work has some features that perpetuate the need for nurses to play communication games in order to influence medical decisions.

These included differences in the scope of decision making between nurses and doctors. Other professionals held assumptions about nurses' work that were largely invisible in written records and to those who visited the ward for short periods. There was also an organisational culture that supported a professional hierarchy, and there was evidence that nurses' complaints could be minimised in order to placate doctors. These features perpetuate the status quo with regard to the way in which healthcare work is carried out. However, drivers for change in nurses' roles arising both from within the nursing profession and from outside it (e.g. opportunities arising from changes in government health policy) lend support to challenging of the status quo. The extent to which real change will be achieved or resisted by participants will determine whether the nurse–doctor game is still needed, or whether it is discarded in favour of an equal contribution and consensus over and agreeing of a care and treatment plan.

Chapter summary box

- Nurses have a historical role that includes management of the care environment as well as care for the patient within it.
- There is a difference between nurses' and doctors' decision making. Treatment prescription is traditionally the remit of the doctor.
- The continual presence of the nurse with the patient supports the generation of a different way of knowing the patient compared with other healthcare professionals.
- Nurses make their narratives known in order to influence and alter medical decisions.
- Several factors influence the communication tactics employed by the nurses to make their narratives known to doctors.

Stop and think

In this chapter the nurse–doctor relationship has been explored together with the communication games that are played in order to make the nurse's narrative known. The following questions ask you to examine the interprofessional relationships in your clinical area and to consider their effect on decision making.

Professionals involved in decision making

- What are the key professional groups involved in ward decision making?
- Does any particular professional group exert control over decision making?
- In what way do they express this control?
- How could the scope of their control be altered so that decision making involves a more equal contribution by professionals and the patient?
- What do doctors understand the role of the nurse to be in your clinical area?
- How does their view of the nurse's role shape their information seeking from nurses' narratives?
- What is the culture of a ward round? Who leads discussion and what is the nurse's contribution? How does the way in which ward rounds are conducted support or inhibit making nurses' narratives known to doctors?

Communication tactics

- Do any informal rules of nurse–doctor communication exist? If so, what are they?
- Do some nurses ignore these rules? If so, what is the effect of this on the nurse–doctor relationship?
- What range of communication tactics are used?
- Which ones are used frequently?
- How are new nursing staff made aware of the nurse–doctor game and how do they learn informal rules of nurse–doctor communication?
- How should pre-registration nursing training prepare students to understand the context of clinical decision making?
- How should pre-registration nursing training be a tool to effect cultural change among nurses with regard to their acceptance or rejection of the nurse–doctor game?

Advocacy

- What circumstances tend to lead to silencing of the nurse's narrative?
- What effect does silencing have on the decisions that are made about the patient?
- Are there any examples in your clinical area where nurses have succeeded in altering medical decisions?
- Analyse some case examples where nurses have altered medical decisions. Identify the communication tactics used and why particular ones were chosen. Compare these cases with other attempts that have failed to alter medical decisions. Can you identify in these case studies any factors that support making narratives known to doctors?
- Are there certain types of medical decision that can be changed by making narratives known and some that typically are not changed?

References

1 Gair G and Hartery T (2001) Medical dominance in multidisciplinary teamwork: a case study of discharge decision making in a geriatric assessment unit. *J Nurs Manage.* **9:** 3–11.

2 Maslin-Prothero S and Masterton A (1999) *Nursing and Politics: power through practice.* Churchill Livingstone, London.

3 Short JA (1995) Has nursing lost its way? *BMJ.* **311:** 303–4.

4 Stein LI (1967) The doctor–nurse game. *Arch Gen Psychiatry.* **16:** 699–703.

5 Hofling C, Brotzman E, Dalrymple S, Graves N and Pierce C (1966) An experimental study in nurse–physician relations. *J Nerv Ment Dis.* **143:** 171–80.

6 Sweet SJ and Norman IJ (1995) The nurse–doctor relationship: a selective literature review. *J Adv Nurs.* **22:** 165–70.

7 Gjerberg E and Kjolsrod L (2001) The doctor–nurse relationship: how easy is it to be a female doctor co-operating with a female nurse? *Soc Sci Med.* **52:** 189–202.

8 Stein LI, Watts DT and Howell T (1990) The doctor–nurse game revisited. *NEJM*. **322:** 546–9.

9 Snelgrove S and Hughes D (2000) Interprofessional relations between doctors and nurses: perspectives from South Wales. *J Adv Nurs*. **31:** 661–7.

10 Adamson BJ, Kenny DT and Wilson-Barnett J (1995) The impact of perceived medical dominance on the workplace satisfaction of Australian and British nurses. *J Adv Nurs*. **21:** 172–83.

11 Castledine G (1998) Clinical specialists in nursing in the UK: 1980s to the present day. In: G Castledine and P McGee (eds) *Advanced and Specialist Nursing Practice*. Blackwell Science, Oxford.

12 Chiarella M (2000) Silence in court: the devaluation of the stories of nurses in the narratives of health law. *Nurs Inquiry*. **7:** 191–9.

13 May C and Fleming C (1997) The professional imagination: narrative and the symbolic boundaries between medicine and nursing. *J Adv Nurs*. **25:** 1094–100.

Chapter 6

Narratives and expert decision makers: creating and using narratives

Introduction • Describing nurses as decision makers: a continuum of decision-making skill • Moving along the continuum: the inexperienced decision maker • Moving along the continuum: the experienced decision maker • Moving along the continuum: the expert decision maker • Conclusion • Stop and think

Introduction

Previous chapters have examined narrative development and its use in making or influencing decisions. Narratives have multiple participants, individual variation in scope and depth that sometimes leads to different versions of knowing the same patient, and different uses. Within the ward, an information hierarchy (individual and team peer review) was a safeguard against competing narratives and engendered a group consensus of knowing each patient. The existence of an information hierarchy implied a typology of nurse decision makers. A popular typology already exists[1] that describes nurses as being on a continuum between novice and expert, and which has shaped nursing curricula in the UK. A different continuum is introduced in this chapter that uses the narrative model as its reference point. Its value lies in offering an explanation of how participant, process and context need to be understood in order to know patients, identify needs, make decisions and influence other decisions. It is not uncommon to hear and read of references made about nurses as expert decision makers, whether in job advertisements or clinical conversations, but how can an expert decision maker be recognised? Furthermore, to what extent is decision-making expertise a static quality of a practitioner? Can it be assumed that a nurse follows a linear trajectory from their initial registration through to some stage in their career at which point they make consistently expert decisions? Or is expertise context dependent, whereby the skill is transferable but has to be adapted to the specific situation that is encountered? In this chapter these questions will be explored. As mentioned in earlier chapters, although I do not claim that the narrative model necessarily explains your area of practice, it could be a useful reference when examining decision making in your own clinical domain.

Describing nurses as decision makers: a continuum of decision-making skill

Nurses' clinical decision making involves people, a process, an outcome and a given setting. Assuming that it is accepted that decision making is a generic skill developed from childhood, it is reasonable to claim that people can apply this skill to a range of different scenarios. When applied to a nursing context, decision-making skill involves the participant utilising what they have within the circumstances of where they are to determine what to do. The combination of person, process and outcome action requires learning different things in order to be able to arrive at the end point of a decision. With regard to narrative-based decision making, this is accomplished via knowing the patient and includes learning how ward teams work, how they use information, how nurses' roles are understood and which stakeholders participate in decision making. The model discussed in Chapter 1 (*see* Figure 1.1) illustrates these domains of learning – person, process, context and outcome – and can be used to explain different types of decision maker according to their skills of narrative creation and use. The types of decision maker associated with this learning can be marked on a three-stage continuum (*see* Figure 6.1) ranging from an inexperienced to an experienced and ultimately an expert decision maker. A summary of the skills that an expert decision maker has developed will be presented next.

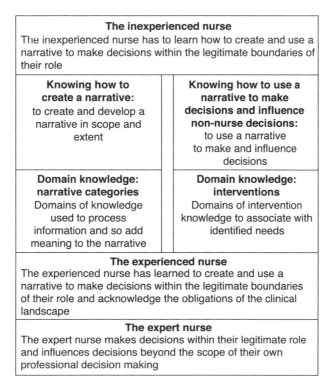

Figure 6.1 Areas of accountability in nursing practice.

Given that the decision-making process has narrative creation and use at its heart, each nurse has to learn how to construct how patients are known and, once this has been attained, they need to know how to use that knowledge to make a decision. Each nurse brings a unique set of knowledge and experiences to decision making, and utilisation of knowledge bases is implied both in narrative development (interpreting and generating narrative category information) and in narrative use (an intervention knowledge base). Decisions are made in a specific setting that shapes how the patient is known and defines boundaries of acceptable outcomes. Healthcare delivery involves multiple participants and incorporates individual and team peer review of the developing narrative. Furthermore, professional, legal and organisational boundaries inform each nurse of their scope of practice and the nature of acceptable decision outcomes. The decision-making process thus takes account of the context, participants and outcome, allowing a nurse to use the narrative in two ways, namely to make a decision within the scope of their legitimate role and to influence non-nursing decisions. An expert decision maker understands the interplay between self, process, context and outcome, has acquired a comprehensive skill set and is experienced in its application. Other nurses have to develop these skills and accrue experience of their application.

An overview of this decision-making skill set is given in Table 6.1 and is linked to aspects of narrative development and use within the wider conceptual framework of participant, process, context and outcome. A nurse's progression along the decision-making skill continuum will be examined next.

Moving along the continuum: the inexperienced decision maker

The trajectory towards expert decision-making practice requires the nurse to know the patient, which involves learning how to create and develop a narrative. This stage characterises the location of the inexperienced decision maker and requires some propositional learning and some learning that can only be gained through experience of local practice. Chapter 1 outlined why nurses have a decision-making role, and explained how this had developed over many decades and how contemporary descriptions of the nurse's role could be understood. This type of learning, drawing on sources that contribute to an awareness of the historical, sociological, professional and legal contexts of nursing practice, allows the nurse to understand their professional identity and determine their roles. These are areas of propositional knowledge. In contrast, experiential knowledge requires the nurse to learn how to create and develop narratives within a specific clinical setting. This includes understanding formal and informal rules of organisational systems and, within the latter, how people work, particularly the ward team.

Understanding different roles

The nurse had at least three different roles (described in Chapter 2) – as nurse carer, care manager and medical assistant. It might be that in other clinical disciplines or other countries, nurses have different or additional roles. Whatever

Table 6.1 The decision-making skill set based on the narrative model

A continuum between:	Creating and developing a narrative	Using a narrative to make decisions	Using a narrative to influence non-nursing decisions	Decision outcome
Inexperienced	*Narrative scope* The inexperienced nurse has partial-scope narratives The inexperienced nurse has partial-scope narratives and limited domain knowledge The inexperienced nurse has to recognise the different roles that a nurse performs in the clinical setting	Limited domain knowledge Decisions made on parts of the narrative	Might be aware of need to challenge as a patient advocate, but has not yet learned the informal rules or tactics to achieve this	Limited to parts of the narrative
⇕				
Experienced	The experienced nurse has full-scope narrative	Decisions made across all three narrative categories and in relation to the patient in a holistic way	Recognises the clinical landscape but tends to operate within its boundaries. Decisions therefore remain within the legitimate scope of the nurse's role	Limited to within the scope of the narrative Satisfies the constraints of the clinical landscape – policy, regulation, more powerful stakeholders
⇕				
Expert	The expert nurse has full-scope narratives	Decisions are made within the legitimate scope of the nurse's role and are made across all three narrative categories giving a holistic view of the patient. The clinical landscape is understood as the narrative is used to shape non-nurse decisions	Recognises the clinical landscape and actively seeks to use the narrative to influence and alter non-nursing decisions where this is deemed necessary	Can extend beyond the scope of the narrative Can challenge the clinical landscape and be a catalyst for change whilst operating within defined boundaries

these are, each nurse has to identify their roles. While propositional knowledge informs them what the role should be, experiential knowledge informs them how that role is interpreted locally. At some stage in their development every nurse compares the ideal with reality and decides which roles have a predominant place in their decision-making practice. Inexperienced nurses, due to their limited exposure to care management, tend towards a care role that typically involves a designated group of patients within the whole ward. Increased experience widens their scope of supervision and so draws them deeper into a range of care management considerations.

The generation of holistic knowledge of the patient requires learning to extend narrative construction beyond using the lens associated with their care role to include information relating to the care management and medical assistant roles. In this way the inexperienced nurse needs to learn to create a full-scope narrative. They also have to understand how their roles and their use of the care record shape information seeking.

Understanding different systems

The inexperienced decision maker has to learn how the system of healthcare is structured at general and local levels. General knowledge includes awareness of the policy framework that shapes the requirements of healthcare delivery. This includes awareness of legal and professional regulation frameworks that shape the scope and standards of practice and establish boundaries of acceptable decision outcomes. Such knowledge facilitates understanding of the context of nurses' work. Locally specific knowledge of the ways of working within the care organisation is also needed. This can only be gained through experience as part of a healthcare team and immersion in the local working culture and practices. These local characteristics are shaped by personalities, interpersonal relationships and team practices.

Inexperienced decision makers also need to learn how formal and informal systems influence the use of information, and what might be considered as 'evidence' to include in the process.

Formal systems: records, rounds and reports

Ward practice has repetitive features that punctuate each working day or week. These are shift handover report, record keeping and medical rounds. Their importance lies in organisational sanction of periodic review and discussion of individual patients. Associated with this is an awareness of how the record system is used to represent the patient and to render them visible within the care process. Within these systems there are ways of recording patient information and rendering visible dominant ways of representing them. The social processes of ward rounds and reports also reveal how different staff groups demonstrate their assumptions about the interprofessional and patient–professional relationships, which by implication mark where the locus of control in decision authority lies. Learning about the location, function and content of nursing records in decision making allows the inexperienced nurse to identify other informal places and information sources that are used in decision making. This develops their appreciation of the role of informal systems in decision making.

Informal systems: personal note sheets and diaries

Informal systems are the 'invisible' practices that complement or compete with formal systems and that can be summed up as 'how things are really done around here'. The difference between verbal and written accounts of patients discussed in Chapter 4 highlighted the role of an oral tradition of care decision making in preference to using a record system at the centre of the process. The peer review system (described earlier as an information hierarchy) was an example of an informal system that was characterised by interpersonal dynamics. It shaped the structure, assumptions and permitted discussion during shift handover reports. Nurses needed to learn what the information hierarchy was and how it was used to guide their practice. Such local knowledge can only be gained during practice, but an examination of it could be included during pre-registration nurse training.

Formal and informal systems relate to the context of narrative development. Nurses also have to learn about the development of narrative content. This relates to narrative scope and depth and implies the use of different knowledge bases.

Understanding narrative domain knowledge

Nurses draw on a range of knowledge bases when processing narrative-category information (nursing, management and medical). Some of this can be learned apart from the clinical setting (propositional knowledge) and is used to establish an atlas of personhood, health and ill health (disease). Continuing study adds detail to the atlas, which typically contains general-level information, but clinical experience offers exposure to a range of variations on general themes. Development of experience facilitates the generation of a richer atlas that incorporates a catalogue of variants of typical cases. Knowledge development in these areas is necessary for nurses to process narrative-category information in order to generate knowledge of patients as individuals rather than as cases aligned to a particular diagnostic label. The curriculum of pre-registration nurse training should outline the atlas of the nurse's role and requisite knowledge bases sufficient to prepare them for practice. However, this is a foundation, and once they are registered, nurses need to add detail to the atlas in relation to a chosen domain of clinical practice. In this way the atlas (narrative-category domain knowledge) is extended by accruing clinical experience. As nurses develop this, so the intellectual capital of the ward team is enhanced and ultimately becomes a resource to guide the practice of other less experienced nurses.

An inexperienced nurse decision maker requires an atlas (domain knowledge relating to general cases) together with experience of variations of general case examples so that narratives are individualised and grounded in the local context. It follows that nurses will have different levels of propositional and experiential knowledge, but decisions need to be made that are holistic, individualised and safe. A tension exists here that is addressed by the ward information hierarchy. Peer review featured highly in the practice of inexperienced nurses, and acted as a safeguard against poor decision-making outcomes. This is one reason why inexperienced nurses have been described as rule driven and reliant on the guidance or instructions of senior staff. However, it is important that inexperienced nurses don't merely copy the practice of experienced staff, which would be ritualistic, but that they understand the processes underpinning decision making so that they can be applied to other situations.

Inexperienced nurses need to learn how to develop full-scope narratives and concurrently develop their domain knowledge through experience of practice. It is one thing to know how to construct and develop a narrative and another to know what to do with that knowledge. A transition therefore has to occur between these two stages, and this makes a distinction between the inexperienced and experienced decision maker.

Moving along the continuum: the experienced decision maker

Nurses need to know how to use the narrative to make decisions. You might recall occasions when a student has witnessed a patient's health crisis and not known what to do, while other staff have acted swiftly with a range of actions to stabilise the situation. A typical example of this occurs in the moments before a patient suffers a cardiac arrest. It is one thing to look at a patient and another to recognise that a problem has become apparent and select the appropriate intervention in response to it. Narrative use involves knowing the patient in order to recognise their needs or problems both within and across categories. Intervention choices are based on generating decision options in relation to identified needs, and these choices imply the existence of an intervention knowledge base, which is an atlas of interventions organised according to the nurse's different roles (care, care management and medical assistant). The process of choosing between decision options takes into account anticipated decision outcomes which imply that the experienced decision maker is aware of the boundaries of their decision making and makes decisions that fall within these.

Experienced decision makers and guidance on decision outcomes

Exposure to different types of intervention with different patients within the same category (for example the dying patient or the patient with emphysema) is learned experientially and is supported by an informal system of peer review. Experienced ward nurses are a key source of intervention information, and the intellectual capital of their accrued wealth of intervention-domain knowledge (propositional and experiential) is integral to developing other nurses' decision-making experience. Through this, inexperienced nurses discuss intervention choices and uncover the locally specific rationales that guide intervention choices in relation to identified needs. Formal and informal systems, such as clinical supervision, reflection on practice and group discussion in report, contribute to the development of each nurse's intervention-domain knowledge.

Nurses' decisions have to fall within the boundary of their legitimate scope of practice and so satisfy legal, organisational, professional, personal and patient requirements. In the UK, nurses have a legal duty of care[2] and standards to maintain under their obligations in the Code of Professional Conduct,[3] which form boundaries to their legitimate scope of practice (discussed further in Chapter 7). Although inexperienced nurses will be aware of these, they require the guidance of experienced staff to ensure that intervention choices will lead to outcomes that fall within the scope of these boundaries.

Progression from inexperienced to experienced decision maker requires skills of narrative development and use. This in turn necessitates parallel development of narrative category and intervention domains of knowledge. Experienced nurses make decisions that fall within the legitimate scope of their role and contribute to the ward information hierarchy and the guidance of less experienced nurses.

Moving along the continuum: the expert decision maker

An expert decision maker takes decision making further in order to influence decisions beyond their legitimate scope of practice. To be able to do this they have to read the clinical landscape and decide to make their narrative visible so that it is acknowledged as a factor to consider in non-nursing decisions. Reading the clinical landscape involves recognising trends and detecting changes in the patient's situation (using the narrative). The decisions made by other participants in the ward environment are considered in relation to their impact on the patient's well-being. Sometimes this includes proposed decisions, and the expert decision maker considers how the narrative would develop if the decision was implemented, and anticipates the outcome. Anticipated narrative development is used to identify whether there is a need to intervene in non-nursing decisions, chiefly medical ones, that affect the patient, and to decide which nurse–doctor communication tactic to use according to their knowledge of interpersonal relationships.

Learning how to become an expert decision maker was commonly spoken of as an experiential process, as on-the-job development that was described as *'learning by Nelly'* and thought to be the *'correct way'* of developing decision-making skills. Experienced decision making could be recognised when a nurse could *'know the patient and can do the care'* by identifying *'what's wrong'* while understanding the patient in a wider context, *'where the patient fits into the whole thing, how it works, and how their illness has impacted on them.'* Expert decision making was recognised when the nurse acted as an advocate for the patient and succeeded in securing a change in decisions which they considered were not in the patient's interest.

A continuum of decision-making skill: oscillations

The development of expert decision-making skills depends on several factors. These include developing propositional and experiential knowledge. The quality of clinical experience and the way in which individual nurses derive benefit from the learning opportunities are more important than the mere passage of time spent in clinical practice. Movement up the continuum involves engagement with the clinical context, its processes, systems and participants, and expert performance is context dependent. The continuum marks a transition from knowing patients and making clinical decisions within the nurse's scope of practice to recognising how others know patients and make decisions that (at times) are not thought to be in the patient's interest. Such decisions can only be effectively challenged when the local clinical landscape is understood. To challenge non-nurse decision makers without knowing which communication tactic is likely to be successful with particular individuals runs the risk of the nurse's narrative being dismissed or rendered invisible.

The decision-making continuum is a convenient means of identifying particular points of skill development. However, once they are performing at an expert level, a nurse might oscillate back and forth between experienced and expert status. There could be different reasons for this, one being the currency of aspects of their knowledge bases (e.g. the latest evidence-based treatments and nursing interventions). If an expert nurse moves to a different ward within the same clinical discipline, there will be a period in which they assimilate the local features of the clinical landscape, principally the informal systems and interpersonal dynamics. It would be anticipated that an expert decision maker would be able to work this out rapidly and operate at an expert level. Even at the margin of an experienced/expert-status decision maker they would be likely to challenge doctors, but the finesse of knowing how to play the nurse–doctor game would need to be attuned to the individuals in that particular ward.

On the other hand, if an expert nurse moved to a new clinical area, their decision-making skills would be transferable but there would be a period of time spent familiarising themselves with the new local clinical landscape and developing the atlas relating to that clinical specialty. It is likely, therefore, that in that particular discipline area they would revert to being an experienced decision maker until these deficits were resolved. Thus there is the possibility of oscillation between expert and experienced decision-maker skill levels.

The invisibility of decision expertise

Nurses' attempts to influence medical decisions were not recorded in their records, and decision-making expertise was acted out rather than written down. Whenever nurses' decision-making practice is invisible in their records they are liable to be seen by doctors and other healthcare professionals as medical assistants and information providers. Given the existing clinical landscape, a case exists for nurses to make their narratives visible so that their expertise is valued by others. Steps in this direction will ultimately challenge the need to play a doctor–nurse game and alter the inter-professional relationships and views of nurses' roles.

The collective resource of decision-making knowledge and experience amounts to the intellectual capital within the ward nursing team. This is often overlooked by non-clinical service managers, who consider wards in terms of economics, systems and targets. However, intellectual capital is a necessary part of regulating decision making and protecting the patient against non-nursing decisions which are thought not to be in their best interest. Proposed changes to the skill mix of the team and to systems of work must anticipate the effect that they will have on patient care. This specifically includes consideration of the effect on the ward information hierarchy, the development of experienced decision-making skills in inexperienced staff and the confidence that patients have in the healthcare team.

Furthermore, loss of experienced and expert staff has to be recognised as a deficit in intellectual capital, and steps need to be taken to maintain and protect team stability. Proposed changes thus need to take a broader view of staff retention and to maximise investments made in staff development.

Organisational change also has to be scrutinised in order to assess the impact that it has on enhancing or inhibiting decision making. An example of this might be changes to local systems, such as altering the place of report and its participants, or moving from written to computer records without examining how this will affect narrative development and use.

The use of temporary staff to cover absences due to sickness and vacant posts needs to be examined in relation to its effect on narrative development, narrative use and intellectual capital. The strongest information hierarchy exists when there is team cohesion and stability. It is unlikely that ad-hoc staff will do much more than contribute to narrative development and have limited time to engage with learning the locally specific formal and informal systems of care delivery. If this is the case, it is likely that the ward team will have to consider how it can make visible its ways of working in order to facilitate cohesive working and draw upon the potential contribution of temporary staff. There is always the possibility that temporary staff might be made to feel like outsiders with regard to the ward culture and, as occurred in the study that underlies this book, concern themselves with the care of individuals according to their own narrative while avoiding the broader scope of management and medical matters.

Decision expertise was largely invisible, particularly in the nursing records, yet it was integral to how nurses actually worked. Ways in which it can be developed need to be considered in order to support staff development and valuing of the ward information hierarchy. Nurses also need to find ways of making this aspect of their work visible so that others recognise its importance in promoting the delivery of safe and effective care and coordinating the contributions of the multi-disciplinary team.

Conclusion

Different levels of decision-making skill can be described using a continuum that spans inexperienced, experienced and expert decision makers. Progression from inexperienced to expert status is via competency development in narrative creation and use both within and beyond the nurse's legitimate scope of practice. It also requires understanding of the broader context of narrative development and use, namely participants, clinical context and outcome. In addition, nurses need to develop their knowledge bases relating to narrative categories and interventions. Although some of this can be propositional knowledge learned through professional education and forming a general and later specialty-based clinical atlas, knowledge derived from experience is also necessary.

Expert and experienced nurses make a vital contribution to the intellectual capital of the ward team, and through the information hierarchy they provide a safeguard against threats to knowing patients, and promote safe and effective decision outcomes. This is often invisible and liable to be overlooked in organisational changes within the ward. In order to safeguard and value decision making and intellectual capital as a central part of nursing work, nurses need to make it visible. The next chapter examines what needs to be made visible and offers a way of demonstrating decision making through an analysis of existing records.

Chapter summary box

- An inexperienced nurse has to learn how to create and use a narrative.
- An experienced nurse decision maker knows how to create and use a narrative and make decisions within their scope of practice.
- An expert nurse decision maker makes decisions within their scope of practice and influences decisions made outside this.
- Decision-making experience and expertise represent intellectual capital within wards.
- Changes in the ward team and organisational design are a threat to the intellectual capital.
- Organisational changes can directly impact on how patients are known and the decisions that are made about them.
- Nurses need to make visible their decision making in order to promote its value as part of their work.

Stop and think

This chapter has provided an explanation of how decision-making expertise is developed. This might assist you as you examine your own description of decision-making expertise. The following questions direct you to explore decision-making expertise in your own clinical area and draw your own conclusions about what it is and how it can be recognised.

A decision-making continuum

- To what extent is the continuum useful for explaining your own level of expertise?
- How would you develop the descriptions of different types of decision maker?
- How are decision makers described in your healthcare organisation's job specifications? How do these differ from the descriptions given in this book?

Expertise and learning

- How do you think decision-making expertise is developed?
- What enhances learning about decision making in the clinical setting?
- How would you describe the intellectual capital within your clinical area?
- What threats exist to preserving the intellectual capital of the ward?
- In what way, if at all, is the intellectual capital of the ward recognised and valued?
- How can the intellectual capital be preserved and developed?

- How can an expected loss of staff (e.g. due to retirement or promotion) be managed so as to minimise a deficit in intellectual capital?
- How would you teach others about informal decision-making processes?
- How would you explain the ward information hierarchy and how it is used in decision making?

Making decision making visible

- What are the formal and informal systems of decision making within your clinical area?
- How does change to the formal system affect informal processes of decision making?
- Is apprenticeship the best model of developing decision-making expertise?
- What role could simulation play in developing decision-making expertise?
- What are the limitations of a simulation of a clinical scenario in developing decision-making expertise?
- How should nursing records be developed to show expertise in decision making?

Atlas – domain knowledge

- What would you define as the minimum atlas needed by a registered nurse?
- How should the atlas be developed during practice?
- How could the learning value of experience be maximised?
- What benchmarks would you use to establish distinctions between inexperienced, experienced and expert decision makers?
- Can there be any short cuts to developing decision-making expertise?
- If you were interviewing applicants for a nursing post, what would you ask about their decision-making skills?
- What role could electronic access to 'knowledge bases' play in replacing the ward information hierarchy?
- How adequate is decision-making skill oscillation as an explanation of the dynamic nature of decision-making status?

References

1 Benner P (1984) *From Novice to Expert: power and excellence in nursing practice.* Addison and Wesley, Menlow Park, California.
2 Department of Health (1979) *The Nurses, Midwives and Health Visitors Act.* HMSO, London.
3 Nursing and Midwifery Council (NMC) (2002) *Guidelines for Records and Record Keeping.* NMC, London.

Chapter 7

Nurses as decision makers: where next?

Introduction • Defining decision making • Demonstrating decisions: what nurses are required to do • Accountability • Nurses' clinical decision making: where next? Professional development implications • Educational implications • Organisational implications • Patient–professional relationship implications • Conclusion • Stop and think

---

Introduction

In previous chapters I have discussed different aspects of nurses' clinical decision making. Their decision-making role developed as a consequence of the effect of intrinsic and extrinsic factors on its contemporary organisational, professional and legally defined scope of practice. The development of expertise, discussed in the previous chapter, demonstrated the need to make nurses' practice visible in order to highlight its value in patient care. The loss of decision-making expertise in clinical areas may not be recognised until problems have occurred. Given that nurses are accountable for their practice, there is a requirement to demonstrate this in clinical records. Although existing record systems do not capture the cognitive work between assessment, plan and intervention choice, there needs to be a means of recording these decision processes and 'capturing' the value of expert decision making and the ward information hierarchy.

The first part of this chapter revisits a definition of decision making and nurses' accountability. Having identified what nurses have to demonstrate, the narrative model is used as a tool to analyse decision making in their records. This could be valuable in teaching or reflective practice situations involving retrospective analysis of decision making. Future developments with regard to nurses' decision making will then be considered.

Defining decision making

Nurses as decision makers can be defined as having an occupational role that is legally defined and organisationally bounded. Development of nursing identity, the scope of their work and the place of its legitimate boundary will continue to be subject to intrinsic factors (e.g. nurses' professionalisation) and extrinsic factors (e.g. social, political, economic and technological developments). When nurses move into autonomous decision making the role becomes a professional and occupational one. In the ward work described in this book, nursing therapy decisions were autonomous, but nurses were also subject to the influence of medical instructions and decision making that made assumptions about their work. These assumptions (about their role as medical assistant) cast nurses as a part of medical decision making, not as fully independent decision makers.

Nurses' decision making involves participants, a process, an outcome and a particular setting, namely the clinical landscape of the ward (*see* Figure 1.1). The nurse uses a narrative-based process to generate decision options and select an intervention, leading to an outcome. This is decision making either about a patient care-related intervention or to influence non-nursing decision making (e.g. medical decisions). Ward nurses work in a team context, so the clinical landscape refers to multiple participants in narrative development and also the working practices, both social and physical (e.g. shift reports, peer review, ward rounds, books, case notes and other records). You will have noticed that the study cited in this book revealed a hierarchical social clinical landscape in which nurses acted as advocates for patients, particularly when considering the impact of medical decision making. Therefore patients were only active in decision making as far as the process was regulated and mediated by nurses. Patients were often involved in understanding the decisions made about them and how they could cooperate in their successful implementation, but were rarely involved in controlling the decision-making process. This implies a decision-making locus of control between patient and professional. Legal and professional obligations of care provision shape nurses' decision-making practice, so can account for why the locus can reside in their domain. The patient, on the other hand, needs to be fully involved in the process and to own any decisions that are made, otherwise they will be relegated to being passive recipients of care and treatment. Service developments that aimed to arrange care services around the patient implied that some features of the existing service design wrapped patients around the processes and choices of hospital staff. Patient-centric care requires more than organisational redesign to make their journey along the care trajectory seamless. It means revisiting the ways in which people work within clinical organisations, and particular understanding of formal and informal systems of work. Formal systems alone were not sufficient to capture how the patient was known and how nursing decisions were made. Informal systems, such as team discussions, use of note sheets and individual peer review, all shaped how the patient was known. To move the locus of decision-making control towards the patient as a full participant in decision making requires these systems to be examined. Furthermore, particular consideration needs to be given to the effect that any such changes will have on narrative development and use. Often formal systems are changed without considering the impact on how people actually work (informal systems) or the effect that this has on knowing patients.

Demonstrating decisions: what nurses are required to do

An examination of nurses' accountability is useful for identifying what nurses are required to demonstrate about their decision making. Figure 7.1 shows areas of nurses' accountability reflecting intrinsic and extrinsic factors that shape the scope and boundary of their work.

The professional regulator is concerned with monitoring whether standards of practice are upheld so that nurses satisfy their legally based duty of care. When working as employees of a health service provider, nurses also have responsi-

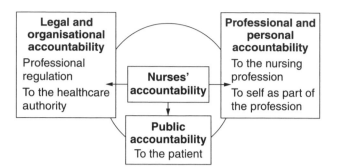

Figure 7.1 Areas of accountability in nursing practice.

bilities to comply with local policies and practices that constitute a visible expression of the organisation's function as a care provider. In addition, nurses represent part of the wider profession and must uphold its standards of practice while at the same time remaining true to their own cultural values and beliefs. Above all, nurses have to be able to demonstrate their accountability to patients. This has been referred to as a nurse's primary accountability, and nurses should expect to be able to demonstrate clinical decisions for the patient's benefit. Given these different forms of accountability, a brief examination of professional guidance (using an example from the UK) allows conclusions to be drawn about how nurses can demonstrate their decisions.

Accountability

Individual decision makers

An assumption in the *Code of Professional Conduct*[1] that each nurse is individually accountable for their decisions is questionable, given that decisions are made in a team context and that nurses are not solely accountable for specific patients over a period of days. The demonstration of decisions is therefore complicated by the multiple participants and the evolving nature of needs identification and decision making.

Department of Health policy requirements also highlight individual accountability for the delivery of care within a framework of clinical governance: *'quality . . . services . . . high standards of care . . . and excellence in clinical care'*.[2] This refers to the quality of decision outcomes and the use of evidence in the process. Aspects of demonstrating proper consideration with regard to the requirements of clinical governance include cost conservation and quality outcomes, and a decision outcome which is measurable and framed in standardised language. This has been argued to enhance the visibility of nurses' work, allowing them to *'seize the opportunities* [of change] *so that nursing's influence on healthcare outcomes will be known'*. A standard nursing language does not exist, nor are there established ways of measuring nurses' decision making, so this claim remains an aspiration of the empowerment of nurses within a wider healthcare team, rather than one of current practice.

Decision outcomes

When referring to decision outcomes, nurses often used descriptions such as 'good' or 'poor'. It is useful to know the meaning of these terms, as this informs what should be included when demonstrating the quality of decisions. Given that inexperienced nurses have to learn how to construct a narrative and identify a patient's needs in order to make decisions, the term 'good' can refer to both the process and the outcome.

A 'good' process can be understood as the nurses' demonstration of their construction of a full-scope narrative with a depth of narrative-category information. Nurses with different levels of experience will be able to demonstrate how they used the narrative to make decisions within their legitimate boundary of practice, or to influence non-nursing decisions. This difference has been reported elsewhere, in a UK-based survey[3] of general ward nurses' clinical decision making in which inexperienced novice nurses were described as *'not knowing their patients'* and made decisions that *'lacked knowledge'*, *'full information'* and the exercise of *'clinical foresight'*. They were also rule driven.

A factor in nurses' acceptance of responsibility for errors, and the implied labelling of these as good or poor, has been associated with their interpretation of the *Code of Professional Conduct*.[1] Demonstration of good, safe and demonstrable decisions by justifying the actions taken requires self-evaluation. It has been argued that a *'feeling of having made the right decision, irrespective of outcome in terms of action'* was a part of the process.[4] A small-scale study of 12 expert nurse decision makers (5 years post registration) supported the use of a problem-solving process and identified a cluster of objective and subjective factors that included a personal philosophy of care as influences on decision making. In the study referred to in this book, one of the subjective factors was the doctor–nurse interaction. There were occasions when nurses had a preferred decision which they considered was in the patient's best interests, but they sometimes had to lay this aside in order to conform with a medical way of knowing the patient. This highlighted the influence of context on judging decision making as good or poor. This has been reported elsewhere in a claim that it was difficult to hold nurses accountable for specific patients, and it was recognised that they sometimes placed *'employers' priorities above patient priorities'*.

Decision process

An organisational requirement for nurses' work to be visible was implied in a discussion of an out-of-court settlement about a case of malpractice that was attributed to a lack of clear, concise documentation (*'the record was silent regarding the charge nurses' response to these reports'*).[5] The outcome of this settlement included a list of recommendations about a verbal communication information hierarchy (team leader, senior staff) through which guidance could be given on decision making. These recommendations also included seven points that nurses needed to record about their decisions (problem identification, communication with others, reports to higher-level managers, any request made for equipment, the response of providers or managers, any recommendations or guidance provided by the team leader, and reassessment of the patient's condition). This list highlights aspects of a decision process that relied on communication, peer review and evaluation, and lends support to the oral tradition that is a part of nurses' narrative-based decision making. The oral tradition was favoured over the use of written records in decision making. This was discussed in Chapter 4, when it was mentioned that nurses reported that records were written to satisfy legal and organisational requirements (reported as avoiding *'being dragged into court'* and *'something we have to do'*). In the UK their legal duty of care is outlined in the Nurses' Act,[6] Rule 18a of which describes their role as having a problem-solving approach to care with decision-making steps (assessment, planning and implementation) and an outcome (evaluation). It implies that nurses have to demonstrate a decision-making process and outcome.

How much to record

Professional regulation exists alongside this legal duty of care to protect the public by ensuring that professional standards are upheld. Three principles underpin professional regulation, namely promoting good practice, preventing poor practice and intervening in unacceptable practice.[7] This was explained by the UKCC as sharing evidence of good practice and working within a framework of the *Code of Professional Conduct*[1] to ensure that care delivery does not put clients at increased risk of harm. However, use of the ill-defined terms 'good' and 'poor' implies that practice is judged by norms within the wider profession. Subsequent *NMC Guidelines for Records and Record Keeping*[8] offered insights into a definition of good practice. Each nurse had to make their own choice ('professional judgement') about when and what to record about their practice, but it had to include a *'full account of the assessment and the care . . . planned'* and *'relevant information'* and *'evidence that you have honoured your duty of care and have taken all reasonable steps to care for the patient or client and that any act or omissions on your part have not compromised their safety in any way'*.

Once again, demonstrating decisions includes an implied problem-solving approach to decision making (assessment, implied problems, care plan and consideration of outcomes). Within this is an assumption that decisions can be easily recognised and a sequential process can be deliberatively represented.

The concept of assessment includes notions of scope (relevant information), but falls short of quantifying the meaning of the term 'full scope' or how this can be recognised when constructing knowledge about a patient. Use of the term 'relevant' also implied an assumption about the usefulness of different categories of information used to identify a patient's problems. This pragmatic approach using a problem-solving sequence, which is a part of Rule 18a (assess, plan, implement and evaluate), almost suggests that the nurse is an information gatherer, that information is available to be gathered, and that it can be accrued in sufficient quantity to allow the diagnosis of a problem. If this is the case, there is an assumption that all assessment information, problems identified and corresponding interventions could be recorded. The narrative section of the record should include notes on the evaluation of goal achievement and problems solved. Nurses' records (in the study referred to throughout this book) did have a problem-solving format. However, even some of those records did not contain a full problem-solving process. Furthermore, it supports the view that at any given recording point one nurse is identified as the sole participant in decision making, when in fact they are part of a care team.

Ways of improving records

Two approaches could be taken to addressing the problems of making decisions visible in nurses' records – first, to impress on nurses their responsibilities with regard to maintaining good records, and second, to revisit record design in order to find ways of capturing how nurses work. The first approach is periodically revisited,[9] and opportunities for the second are available wherever provider organisations sanction development of their record systems. The advent of a national record system as a 'one-size-fits-all' approach is a threat to this second option, as there is no guarantee that it will improve on existing attitudes towards care record usage in decision making. Furthermore, it remains to be seen how developments such as an electronic national care record can align record keeping to nurses' ways of working and capture the processes involved. Whatever the failings of the existing record systems, nurses have to demonstrate their accountability. The record system therefore needs to be reviewed to determine how it can be developed to capture nurses' practice.

The narrative decision-making model, if it represents how decisions are made, could offer a framework to be incorporated in the redesign of records. Developments in this area could make nurses' roles and information categories visible, formalise judgements as information processing, and identify decision options and decisions taken. The narrative model could also be useful for analysing nurses' decisions in existing care records.

Using the narrative model to demonstrate decision making

Use of the narrative decision-making model can facilitate giving a response to the meaning of the statement in professional guidance that a nurse has *'taken all reasonable steps to care for the patient or client'*. Formerly, under the UKCC,[10] nurses had to *'demonstrate their properly considered clinical decisions'*, and *'having taken all reasonable steps'* can be interpreted as recording decision making in such a way that it satisfies the range of a nurse's accountability (legal, regulatory, professional and personal, and to the patient) and captures the real-world processes of clinical decision making. The narrative model can be a useful tool to identify first the processes involved (narrative creation and development), and second, how the narrative (knowing the patient) is used to make nursing decisions or influence other decisions. The following example outlines a way in which this model could be used within clinical supervision, clinical teaching or reflective practice to examine decision making.

The different parts of the narrative model can be transposed into a table, as shown in Table 7.1. This table has column headings of information type, narrative category, judgements within categories, global judgements of how the patient is known and statements of movement along the care trajectory as a 'trajectory marker'. These columns represent narrative development. The last four columns represent narrative use and include problems identified, intervention options, decisions made and decision outcome. The text of the record is divided into chunks and inserted into the first two columns, the first being an index number relating to each data chunk. The table could also be used to analyse a transcript of a shift report so that written and verbal accounts of the same patient could be compared.

Table 7.1 The narrative decision model transposed into a table to be used to analyse transcripts of nurses' records

	Narrative data		Narrative creation					Narrative use			
Data chunk	*Text of narrative*		*Information*	*Narrative category*	*Judgements (in categories)*	*Judgements (global)*	*Trajectory marker*	*Problems identified*	*Intervention option*	*Decision made*	*Decision outcome*
1											
2											
3											
4											

An analysis of a brief text example using this table format is shown in Table 7.2. In this analysis the patient is represented as a medical case requiring treatment. The nurse's role is cast as supporting medical contribution, and chiefly marks the stage of the patient's progression along the care trajectory. Although there are hints of a nurse–patient discussion, nothing was recorded about other needs that the patient might have or of any nursing actions that were taken. Similarly, there were hints of using the nursing lens and demonstrating that the patient was known as an individual within the healthcare process. In summary, this brief analysis portrays the patient as a medical case and the nurse's role as that of a medical assistant and care manager. As a result, other nursing work is rendered invisible.

This table is divided into columns which indicate the overall process of narrative creation and use leading to the decisions made. The columns identify various aspects of each stage.

The text used in this analysis is taken from a nursing record:

> Reason for admission: *To see the doctors for IV methylprednisolone.*
> Final diagnosis: *?Retrobulbar neuritis.*
> Past medical history: *Had some tests but doesn't know what.*
> History: *Had an episode of numbness and altered sensation up to her waist, which has resolved. Four days ago she developed blurred vision in the left eye.*

Nurses' clinical decision making: where next?

Nurses have to make their decision making accountable for a number of reasons. Demonstrating narrative-based decision making has implications in several areas. These include professional development considerations of nurses as decision makers, educational implications with regard to the process of nurses' decision making and development of expertise, and organisational implications with regard to the means of recording nurses' work and judging the quality of decision

Table 7.2 An example of the use of the analytical table to analyse a nursing record excerpt

	Narrative data	Narrative creation				Narrative use				
Data chunk	Text of narrative	Information	Narrative category	Judgements (in categories)	Judgements (global)	Trajectory marker	Problems identified	Intervention option	Decision made	Decision outcome
1	Reason for admission: *To see the doctors for IV methylprednisolone*	Treatment	Medical		A medical case waiting to see a doctor	To see doctor	Needing treatment		Needs medical intervention	
2	Final diagnosis: *?Retrobulbar neuritis*	Diagnosis	Medical		Diagnosis		Potential diagnosis			
3	Past medical history: *Had some tests but doesn't know what*	Investigation	Nursing		Individual					
4	History: *Had an episode of numbness and altered sensation up to her waist, which has resolved. Four days ago she developed blurred vision in the left eye*	Patient report – limbs Patient report – vision	Nursing	Health stability Health change	Individual		Blurred vision			

outcomes. Patient–professional relationships in participation in and control of decision making constitute a further area of development.

Professional development implications

There are good reasons to support the case for intrinsic development of the nurse's role as a decision maker. Nurses are well situated to coordinate care and extend the scope of their role to offer a broader contribution to patient care. This can include moves into what was formerly the territory of other professionals, and has led to questions of whether nurses are becoming 'mini doctors' or 'maxi nurses'. Economic and organisational expediency might move professional development in this direction as new ways are considered to efficiently deploy limited medical staff resources. The scope of nurses' decision making is to a large extent bounded by extrinsic factors. Nurses could take advantage of existing resource pressures on healthcare organisations and pursue a path towards autonomous practice. If they do this they will need to be able to identify the nature of extrinsic factors that shape their role and the mechanisms by which they establish a boundary to their legitimate scope of practice. Awareness of this could be used to inform their professional development strategies.

Ways of representing nursing work also include the terminology used. At present a universally agreed nursing vocabulary does not exist. Such a nomen-clature could be useful, especially when developing consistent coding systems that could be used to identify parts of the decision process. However, national health services are a collection of many local services that have their own particular social and organisational subculture. It is likely that these services employ different terms to describe their practice, and until these are known the establishment of an (inter)national vocabulary system will be limited.

Educational implications

Traditionally the development of decision-making skill has been learned 'on the job' through clinical experience. It is possible to use the narrative model to identify key steps in decision making and to find ways of developing related learning in classroom rather than clinical settings. It should be possible to use the conceptual framework to explain decision making and the narrative model (for example) to examine details of the processes involved. Given this model, pre-registration nurses could be guided to examine the development of their own decision-making skills, while their clinical mentors could use it as a reference to identify within the local setting where and how these skills can be developed. The continuum of decision-making expertise is also useful for registered staff to use in reflective practice and self-assessment for decision-making skill and goal setting for professional development.

Organisational implications

Those responsible for service provision need to consider how effective their record systems are in representing nurses' work, particularly decision making, and especially in relation to the extent that these systems facilitate demonstration of accountability in decision making. Before any organisational change such as the introduction of a new record system, the implications for the formal and informal systems need to be thought through with a view to anticipating the effect that the change is likely to have on patient care. Organisational change also has to take account of the impact that it might have on team stability, cohesion and the intellectual capital of the ward, as these all affect the decision-making process.

Modern health services are target driven and have to be accountable to patients. The quality of decision outcomes is a relevant measure that forms a useful starting point for examining the process used. Moves to define the quality of decision outcomes are also useful for establishing collaboration between expert practitioners and expert patients.

Patient–professional relationship implications

The participation of patients in the decisions that are made about them can frequently be limited. The locus of control in decision making is not necessarily fixed, and can alter, for example as a result of policy measures that espouse full patient participation in shared decision making. The locus of control is likely to alter according to the preferences of each individual patient, their health status and their interaction with staff. Demonstration of nurses' decisions needs to account for these differences and display where the locus of decision making predominantly lies. This could be useful for offering a response to policy moves that insist on a single approach to decision making based on the assumption that the patient wishes to, or is capable of, making and owning decisions about their own health needs.

Conclusion

Nurses' decision making is complex. To suggest that nurses just provide care and equate this to task performance is to overlook a central feature of their work. There is therefore a need to make nurses' decision making visible, and this requires understanding of the processes involved and use of a terminology that makes these meaningful. The value of championing nurses' decision-making work is ultimately for the patient's benefit, although it also offers advantages for developing professional identity. We have seen that the clinical landscape influences the decisions made about patients, and that this can be dominated by the medical model and doctors. Nurses are with the patient for 24 hours a day, and their way of knowing the patient can, if they have a full-scope narrative, be holistic and generate an understanding of the patient's experience as they progress though the experience of clinical care and treatment. It is the strength that comes through knowing patients in this way that makes it necessary to challenge any moves that decentre the focus of healthcare delivery away from the patient as an individual – be it other professionals, policies or organisational change.

Chapter summary box

- Nurses have a range of accountabilities.
- Written records are the primary source of demonstrating nurses' work.
- Written records do not capture all that nurses do, and when these records are redesigned, consideration needs to be given to methods of capturing the scope of nurses' decision-making work.
- The narrative model can be used to analyse existing records in order to demonstrate some aspects of nurses' decision making.
- Nurses are in a unique position of knowing patients on account of their 24-hour presence with them on the ward.
- Nurses' use of their narratives is necessary to challenge any moves that decentre the patient and their needs from the focus of healthcare delivery.

Stop and think

In this chapter, ways and implications of demonstrating decisions have been discussed. The final 'stop and think' questions ask you to look ahead to work out what the immediate implications are for yourself and your decision-making practice.

Demonstrating decisions

- Select a sample of your own record keeping and analyse it using the table given in this chapter to evaluate how you have represented the patient and the decisions that you have made concerning them (you might need to seek local organisational approval to use an excerpt from a formal record).
- Consider your findings and explore what you could have written and did not, and how, if it had been included, this would have altered the representation and decisions made about the patient.

Challenging the influence of the clinical landscape

- Consider a series of your written records and try to identify other factors in the clinical landscape that have influenced the decision-making process.
- Are these explicit in the records or do they spring to mind when you are reading through them?
- If influences in the clinical landscape are not explicit, to what extent should these be recorded to show how a decision was shaped?
- Would the threat of a complaint against the nursing team alter the content of what was written about the patient?

- If the content is different, in what way would it be so?
- Can you think of examples where the preferred decision made about the patient was altered to one influenced by someone else?
- If you can, examine these as case studies to determine what you would do differently to counter the identified influences.
- Are there any implications for developing your own practice so that you can be confident of success in challenging moves that, according to your knowledge of the patient, would decentre them from the focus of care delivery? What are those implications?

References

1 United Kingdom Central Council (UKCC) (1992) *Code of Professional Conduct.* UKCC, London.

2 Department of Health (1998) *Information for Health.* The Stationery Office, London.

3 Gurbutt R (2005) *Demonstrating nurses' clinical decision making.* PhD thesis. University of Central Lancashire, Preston.

4 Maas ML (1998) Structure and process constraints on nursing accountability. *Outcomes Manage Nurs Pract.* **2:** 51–3.

5 Mahlmeister L and Koniak-Griffin D (1999) Professional accountability and legal liability for the team leader and charge nurse. *J Obstet Gynecol Neonatal Nurs.* **28:** 300–9.

6 Great Britain (1979) *The Nurses, Midwives and Health Visitors Act.* HMSO, London.

7 United Kingdom Central Council (UKCC) (2001) *Professional Self-Regulation and Clinical Governance.* UKCC, London.

8 Nursing and Midwifery Council (NMC) (2002) *Guidelines for Records and Record Keeping.* NMC, London.

9 The Health Service Ombudsman.

10 United Kingdom Central Council (UKCC) (1993) *Standards for Records and Record Keeping.* UKCC, London.

Suggested lesson plans

The following module description and learning units are offered as a possible way of using the text as a focus for decision-making study. The module could be adopted in its entirety, or alternatively it could form learning units that are embedded in other programmes of study.

Module description

Module title	Clinical decision making

Module aims

The aims of this module are to:

- examine the role of nurses as decision makers
- examine a narrative explanation of real-world decision making
- examine local clinical practice and consider decision making in relation to the narrative-based decision-making model
- examine the process, context, outcome and participants in decision making
- examine decision makers and decision expertise
- examine decision-making accountability.

Module content

The module comprises seven learning units. Each one focuses on an aspect of real-world decision making and links examination of published evidence and policy to the student's own area of practice.

Learning Unit 1 Setting the scene: the clinical landscape of decision making
Learning Unit 2 Making clinical decisions: a model of nurses' decision-making
Learning Unit 3 The narratives that nurses generate: ways of knowing the patient
Learning Unit 4 Demonstrating narratives: differences between verbal and written narratives
Learning Unit 5 The games nurses play: making narratives known to doctors
Learning Unit 6 Narratives and expert decision makers: creating and using narratives
Learning Unit 7 Nurses as decision makers: where next?

Skill development

The development of a range of skills forms part of the module activities, including developing communication skills (group discussion and learning feedback), IT (literature searching), problem solving (discussing solutions to dilemmas such as record keeping) and managing one's own learning (planning what to study and using resources effectively). These will support the professional practice and participation in a range of clinical leadership and healthcare delivery activities.

Teaching and learning strategy

The module will be delivered using a range of learning and teaching strategies designed to meet the learning outcomes. There will be a combination of formal teaching, blended learning (e.g. Web-based materials), supplementary reading to extend learning, group work, reflection and discussion exercises that facilitate students' development of analysis and review of theory and practice.

Students will prepare short talks based on their reflective work and extension exercises that examine aspects of workplace decision making. Each session includes a period of group feedback on extension learning and reflections from practice.

Students will keep a reflective diary to help to inform their professional development plan.

Learning outcomes

On successful completion of this module a student will be able to:

1	Explain the role of nurses as decision makers and factors that have shaped its development
2	Explain the scope of decision-making enquiry in their chosen clinical field
3	Evaluate published evidence about nurses' real-world decision making and evaluate the adequacy of theoretical models to explain practice in the student's clinical area
4	Describe local processes involved in decision making
5	Evaluate the role and contribution of record keeping in decision making
6	Identify the boundaries of nurses' decision making and how non-nursing decisions are influenced
7	Examine concepts of experienced and expert decision makers and decision making

Assessment of learning
Assignment
The assignment options offer students the opportunity either to examine literature-based accounts of decision making in a chosen area of practice, or to examine and analyse a real-world decision made in their own practice.

The assignment can be adapted to different levels of academic assessment through substitution of different terms in the guidance given (e.g. describe, synthesise, analyse, critically analyse).

Module pass requirements
Completion of the assignment to the agreed minimum threshold mark for a pass. The weighting of the assignment is 100%.

Learning units

Learning Unit 1 Setting the scene: the clinical landscape of decision making

Lesson aims
1 Examine the historical development of the role of the nurse.
2 Examine the legal, professional and organisational requirements for nurses' practice as decision makers.

Text reference – Chapter 1.

Learning outcomes – 1 and 2.

	Learning content	*Staff contribution*	*Student activity*	*Learning resources*
1	Defining the role of the nurse.	Introduce the subject by discussion, perhaps a popular press depiction of nursing practice.	Student group discussion – create a taxonomy of nurses' work. Summarise the taxonomy as a paragraph defining 'nurse' and the nurse's role.	Seek a range of definitions of 'nurse' in texts/ journals/policy documents. Compare and contrast these.
2	Professional and policy views of the nurse's role.	Examine contemporary definitions of the nurse's role.	Examine abstracts of statements about the legal and professional role of the nurse in health policy documents and professional guidance.	For example, Nursing and Midwifery Council (2002) *Code of Professional Conduct*, and the Nurses Act (1988).

3	Factors that have shaped the role of nurses as decision makers.	Identify historical and sociological accounts of nursing development. Draw out political, economic, social, educational and professional factors that have shaped the definition of the nurse's role.	Explain how this role has changed over a chosen period of time (e.g. 100 years).	Refer to articles/ texts on nursing history.
4	The clinical landscape – the context of nurse decision making.	Define and examine the features of the clinical landscape in a contemporary clinical setting (e.g. a ward): • participants • organisational design and culture • technological factors • health policy.	Students discuss and write on a flipchart/ whiteboard all the factors that they can identify as parts of the clinical landscape. Students try to group these into categories to formulate a summary explanation of the clinical landscape.	Whiteboard. Flipchart.
5	Summary.	Conclude the learning unit with a review of the nurse's role as a decision maker and its context.	1 Select an area for further study and pre-reading for next learning unit (Chapter 2). 2 Make notes in a personal reflective diary of the type and number of decisions that you make during a shift. Note the different types of decision made by different grades of nurse.	

Learning unit summary
By the end of this learning unit students will have examined the role of the nurse as a decision maker, and factors which shape the development of that role, and will have established through reference to key documents a contemporary definition of the scope of practice of the nurse's role as a decision maker.

Suggested areas for further study	
1	*The history of nursing practice* Examine literature on the history of nursing with a view to identifying references made about the nurse's role as medical assistant and support of medical decision making. Which developments in nursing practice have marked a move towards making nursing decisions in contrast to supporting medical decision making?
2	*The scope of existing enquiry in a chosen area of practice* Undertake a literature search of nurse decision making in your chosen discipline area over the past 20 years. Identify the number of papers that have the keywords 'decision making' and 'nurse' and from the ones that you retrieve, summarise the types of study that have been undertaken (the methodological approach), the research questions that have been asked and the findings/claims that are made about nurses' decision making. What can you identify about the need for further study of nurses' decision making?
3	*Doctors' views of nurses and their work* Examine medical literature (e.g. the *British Medical Journal*) for articles that discuss nurses' roles, and identify how these are portrayed in terms of educational levels, decision authority and clinical activities. Compare your findings with current policy statements and professional guidance about the nurse's role.

Learning Unit 2 Making clinical decisions: a model of nurses' decision-making

Lesson aims

1 Examine the types of decisions that nurses make and which nurses make these decisions.

2 Examine the number of nursing decisions that are made during a period of duty.

3 Examine how decisions are made.

4 Examine the theoretical explanations of decision making.

Text reference – Chapter 2.

Learning outcomes – 1, 2, 3 and 4.

	Learning content	Staff contribution	Student exercises	Learning resources
1	Introduction.	Having established the role and context of nurses as decision makers, the focus of study moves on to how decisions are made.	1 Recap learning and feedback from previous learning unit. 2 Students give feedback on their findings from their further study. 3 Selected students report back on the types and number of decisions made in practice.	
2	The decisions that nurses make.	Refer to selected literature and highlight the range of decisions reported that nurses make. Compare literature-based accounts with those generated by students.	1 Group exercise to develop a description of the scope, types and frequency of decisions made in practice. 2 Group work to categorise the decisions.	Reference to different types of decisions reported in recent nursing literature.

3	Do different nurses make different decisions?	Examine the different responsibilities that different types/grades of nurse have and the common responsibilities that all nurses have. Examine the links between nurses' decisions and types of nurse decision makers. Refer to examples of role descriptions.	1 Discussion about the differences in decisions made by different designations of nurse. 2 Examine a selection of nursing role descriptions and identify the ways in which decision making is a part of the role and differs between different grades of nurse.	Reference to role descriptions of staff nurses, junior sisters/ charge nurses, senior sisters/ charge nurses, ward specialist nurses, clinical managers.
4	How decisions are made – the narrative model as a way of explaining how patients are known.	Introduce students to a descriptive model of decision making and identify the participants, processes and information processing. Discuss the conceptual lens as a means of explaining how role and information seeking are related.	Referral to Chapter 2 (narrative model). 1 Compare the model with experience of local practice, to identify similarities and differences. 2 Discuss any differences and how these impact on representing how the patient is known.	Reference to papers offering different theories of nurses' real-world decision making.
5	Theoretical explanations of decision making.	Introduce students to prescriptive and descriptive explanations of decision making.	Discuss the advantages and disadvantages of the two main theoretical explanations of decision making in connection with learning how to make decisions and represent patients and their needs.	Refer to selected decision-making review articles on prescriptive and descriptive decision making.

| 6 | Summary. | Conclude the learning unit with a review of different ways of explaining decision making. Identify further learning in selected areas of theoretical knowledge and practice. | 1 Decide an area for further study and pre-reading for next learning unit (Chapter 3).

2 Record in a personal reflective diary some examples of how different patients are known and described in the chosen clinical area. | |

Learning unit summary

By the end of this learning unit students will have examined the scope and types of decisions that nurses make and the differences between different grades of nurse. The real world of clinical practice will have been discussed in order to estimate the number of decisions made during a typical period of duty. The process of decision making will have been examined, including the narrative model (Chapter 2) which is used as a reference to focus discussion about the participants, processes in knowing patients and making decisions. This will have included consideration of role and the conceptual lens in information seeking.

Suggested areas for further study

1	*Reflection on observed or personal practice* Observe/reflect on a shift spent in a clinical area and identify the range of decisions made, and which decisions are made most frequently, and compare these with the description of a nurse's decision-making role (Learning Unit 1). Do nurses need to make all of these decisions? Should some decisions be delegated to non-nurses? Are there other decisions that nurses could make but currently do not?
2	*Explaining local decision making* Discuss with different members of the nursing team in your chosen clinical area how they think their decisions are made. Reflect on the accrued responses and draft a tentative description of the real-world decision-making practice of the local nursing team. Consider to what extent this description is useful for identifying the information processes involved. Is there anything missing? Is this description sufficiently explicit to explain to a student how to make decisions?
3	*Decision processes: focus on report – where does it occur, what is communicated and how is this information used?* Examine the literature on the nursing report and identify different accounts of its purpose, place and content. Consider how different types of report affect the construction of a narrative of the patient.

Learning Unit 3 The narratives that nurses generate: ways of knowing the patient

Lesson aims

1 Examine different ways in which the patient is known.
2 Examine narrative scope and depth.
3 Examine the processes of narrative development – handover report.
4 Examine how different staff contributions and judgements shape how a patient is known.

Text reference – Chapter 3.

Learning outcomes – 3 and 4.

	Learning content	Staff contribution	Student exercises	Learning resources
1	Introduction.	Having examined how decisions are made using the narrative model, attention is now directed towards how the narrative can be used to explain how patients are known.	1 Recap learning and feedback from previous learning unit and feedback from further study. 2 Selected students give feedback on their reflective accounts of how patients are described and known in their clinical area.	
2	How much is known about the patient?	Examining the meaning of 'knowing the patient'.	Commencing with individual reflections on practice-based examples of differences in knowing patients, students consider the extent to which narrative scope and depth can be used to explain these differences.	Peer-reviewed literature that discusses concepts of 'knowing' patients.

3	How much is enough knowledge about a patient?	Introduce the concept of narrative scope and depth. Discuss the variation between staff in knowing patients and why this might be.	1 Discuss whether knowledge about a patient can be summarised as 'enough' or 'not enough'. 2 Discuss what the criteria should be to quantify 'sufficient knowledge' about a patient needed to make decisions.	Chapter 3.
4	What do we tell others? Handover report.	Examine the process of nursing report.	1 Reflect on and discuss the content, place and process of handover report. 2 Using a whiteboard, generate a summary of how reports are performed in different clinical areas. Examine the similarities and differences, and consider how these shape knowing patients.	Chapter 3. Peer-reviewed papers about the role of handover report.
5	How are patients described? Judgements.	Examine the different examples of judgements made about patients (Chapter 3). Explore how information is processed to offer summary representations of knowing patients.	1 Discuss/reflect on local ways of describing patients. 2 Examine cases of patients being described in ways that portray them as objects rather than as people, and analyse why this is so.	Reflective accounts of clinical practice.

| 6 | Summary. | Conclude the learning unit with a review of possible ways of knowing patients and the ways in which global judgements are used to summarise how patients are known. | 1 Decide on an area for further study and pre-reading for the next learning unit (Chapter 4).

 2 Obtain (assuming permission is given) an anonymised excerpt from a nursing record of patient care to use in classroom discussion. | |

Learning unit summary

By the end of this learning unit students will have examined ways of knowing patients, the scope and depth of a narrative, the report process and judgements used to summarise how patients are known.

Suggested areas for further study

1	*Knowing patients* Examine the nursing literature for accounts of 'knowing' patients. Identify how knowing patients is or is not valued and the variation in explanations of the meaning of 'knowing' patients.
2	*Judgement* Conduct a literature search in the linked areas of 'information processing' and 'nurse decision making'. Search for the use of the term 'judgement' within nursing decision-making papers and identify how this term can have different meanings.
3	*Report* Observe a nursing shift handover report. Identify where it occurs, the participants, the information given and its sequence, the documents used and the interactions that take place. Reflect on your observations and consider what other ways of 'doing report' might be more effective in communicating about knowing patients and their needs. Consider the implications of altering the local method of report for the way in which patients are known by the nursing team.

Learning Unit 4 Demonstrating narratives: differences between verbal and written narratives

Lesson aims

1 Examine the design of nursing records.
2 Examine the differences between verbal and written accounts of patients.
3 Examine the use of informal records in wards.
4 Explore the implications of omitting information from formal nursing records.

Text reference – Chapter 4.

Learning outcomes – 4 and 5.

	Learning content	*Staff contribution*	*Student exercises*	*Learning resources*
1	Introduction.	Having examined the narrative explanation of knowing patients, attention is directed towards comparing and identifying differences between written and verbal accounts of the patient.	1 Recap learning and feedback from previous learning unit. 2 Students give feedback on their findings of their further study about the use of the term 'judgement' in clinical decision making.	
2	How is the account about a patient and their care recorded?	Present the nursing process as a problem-solving approach to documenting nursing work. Examine examples of nurses' records. Discuss what would constitute the ideal record for supporting clinical decision making.	1 Class members present their examples of anonymised nursing records. 2 Compare the different formats of representing the patient, the categories of information recorded and points where decisions are identified.	Professional guidance. Peer-reviewed literature about the use of the nursing process.

3	Differences between what is said and what is written.	Discuss problems with record keeping – make references to legal cases where nursing records have been criticised (e.g. for omission).	1 Compare what is said during report with what is written about a patient, and try to identify the differences and their implications of knowing the patient. 2 Discuss what is often omitted from written records.	Health service ombudsman reports.
4	Informal records.	Discuss the use of a range of informal records (note sheets, diaries, office whiteboards) and their function as information sources used in decision making.	1 Examine local examples of informal records. Consider why these are used and why they are not superseded by a single record. 2 Consider how the introduction of electronic healthcare records will impact on the use of informal paper records in wards.	Examples of informal records. Chapter 4 – nurses' note sheets.

| 5 | Summary. | Conclude the learning unit with a review of the legal requirements with regard to documenting care, and the problems of capturing the scope of information seeking and processing in the record. Include the problem of formal and informal records when examining complaints against nurses' care decisions. | 1 Decide on an area for further study and pre-reading for the next learning unit (Chapter 5).

2 Make notes in your reflective diary about the different inter-professional relationships in the ward. | |

Learning unit summary

By the end of this learning unit students will have examined the differences between written and verbal accounts of the patient, the use of informal records and the legal implications of record keeping.

Suggested areas for further study

1	*Literature search* Examine the legal requirements concerning nurses' record keeping and the specific guidance of the professional regulating body on what nurses should record. Examine a case of clinical negligence (look for reports published by the professional body) and identify the use of the record in explaining the nurse's actions, noting any criticisms that were raised about it. What can be learned from analysis of a clinical negligence case about recording practice? How can a nurse defend their practice if the formal record omits some information?
2	*Informal records* Identify the range of informal records used in the ward. How are these used in the process of decision making, what types of information do they contain and what would happen if these records were removed from use?
3	*Verbal narratives* Consider the verbal narrative – that is, the information that is held in a nurse's memory about a patient. How can the full range of information that nurses discuss be captured in the written record? Or is this not possible?

Learning Unit 5 The games nurses play: making narratives known to doctors

Lesson aims

1 Examine the nurse–doctor relationship.
2 Examine explanations of differences in nursing and medical decision making.
3 Examine how nurses can play communication games in order to influence medical decisions.

Text reference – Chapter 5.

Learning outcomes – 2 and 5.

	Learning content	*Staff contribution*	*Student exercises*	*Learning resources*
1	Introduction.	Having examined how decisions are made and recorded, attention is directed to the ways in which nurses influence (medical) decisions that lie outside their legitimate scope of practice.	1 Recap learning and feedback from previous learning unit. 2 Students give feedback on their findings from their further study.	
2	Nurse–doctor relationships.	Consider the context of acute care delivery and the organisational, professional, social, educational and policy factors that support particular roles (legitimate scope of practice) and behaviour (hegemony).	1 Feed back reflections on the nature of inter-professional relationships within wards. 2 Examine the reasons why differences in decision authority and organisational/ positional power exist in the workplace.	Literature reporting on the nurse–doctor game.

3	Communication tactics.	Discuss the different tactics used in the nurse–doctor game. Examine the rise in patient involvement in decision making as a consequence of a move to patient-centred services.	Discuss and evaluate how the game is played (if at all) and how it might be removed from nurse–doctor interactions in hospital wards.	Policy documents on patient-centred services and advocacy services.
4	Just knowing.	Discuss the concept of an 'intuitive' feeling that a problem exists and how nurses might explain this.	1 Explore explanations of intuitive or 'gut feelings' about a patient and their needs. 2 Examine relevant literature on the value of intuition as an 'art' in nurses' decision-making practice.	Literature on the nature of intuition and its value in clinical practice.
5	Summary.	Conclude the learning unit with a review of the clinical landscape and the differences in decision authority concerning patient care and care management.	1 Decide on an area for further study and pre-reading for the next learning unit (Chapter 6). 2 Make notes in your reflective diary about nurses whom you consider to be expert decision makers. Describe expertise and how it is demonstrated in the practice of these nurses.	

Learning unit summary
By the end of this learning unit students will have examined the nature of inter-professional relationships in the ward, and differences in decision-making authority. The learning unit will also have included an exploration of the ways in which nurses seek to alter or challenge medical decisions. Consideration will also have been given to nurses' intuitive knowledge that a patient problem exists and how this can be understood and used to alter medical decisions.

Suggested areas for further study	
1	*Literature search* Examine the literature on the nurse–doctor game and consider how this relates to hegemony in the clinical workplace. What impact does playing the nurse–doctor game have on the way in which nurses and their work are represented? Given the prevalence of the medical model in the design of care services, to what extent should nursing practice, and its limits, be defined by the medical profession?
2	*Game playing* Try to find examples of clinical areas where the nurse–doctor game is and is not played. Compare these and seek to identify similarities and differences. What reasons can you suggest to account for the need for game playing in one area and not the other?
3	*Organisational design* Examine the organisational context of care delivery and identify factors that empower/support nurses in making a contribution or challenge to non-nursing decisions. In a similar way, identify factors which you consider inhibit contributing to or challenging non-nursing decisions. Why do these factors exist and can they be minimised? Are there any reasons to support the continued existence of these empowering/resistance factors?

Learning Unit 6 Narratives and expert decision makers: creating and using narratives

Lesson aims

1 Examine descriptions of nurses as inexperienced, experienced and expert decision makers.
2 Examine decision-making skills.
3 Explore the concept of intellectual capital.
4 Examine how expertise can be learned or developed.

Text reference – Chapter 6.

Learning outcomes – 7.

	Learning content	Staff contribution	Student contribution	Learning resources
1	Introduction.	Having examined how interprofessional realtionships shape decision making, attention is now turned to nurses as expert decision makers.	1 Recap learning and feedback from previous learning unit. 2 Students give feedback on the notes made in their reflective diaries about decision-making expertise.	
2	What is decision-making expertise?	Examine the concept of a decision-making skills continuum ranging from inexperienced to expert decision maker.	1 Discuss, referring to the narrative model, how understanding roles, domain knowledge and systems knowledge influence skill development. 2 Discuss the elements necessary for a knowledge and skills framework to be developed. Compare this with existing frameworks (NHS KSF).	Chapter 6. NHS Knowledge and Skills Framework (NHS KSF).

3	Intellectual capital.	The knowledge and skills that a nurse possesses can be described as intellectual capital. Examine the effects of organisational change on team stability, and the impact on intellectual capital. Explore how this might affect the decisions made about patients.	1 Using the narrative model, identify points where narrative development and use draw upon the intellectual capital of the ward team and role models. 2 Determine the effect of loss of intellectual capital at these points on decision process and outcome.	Chapter 6.
4	Expert decision makers and role descriptions.	Is decision-making skill explicitly sought in role descriptions for nursing jobs? Examine a range of role descriptions to develop an answer to questions of the extent of invisibility of decision making in the nurse's role. If the term 'expert nurse' is used, how is this understood within the role descriptions examined?	1 Examine a range of role descriptions and abstract information indicating that decision making is recognised as part of the nurse's role. 2 Examine the implicit assumptions about how nurses make decisions, how they are recognised and how they can be evaluated as expert decisions.	Job descriptions/ specifications.

5	Leaning to be an expert decision maker.	Is there a 'best' method of developing decision-making expertise? Examine educational approaches to developing decision-making skills using vignettes, simulations and practice-based learning. Discuss the usefulness of reflection and critical incident analysis.	1 Group discussion about approaches to learning how to make clinical decisions in practice. 2 Explore what can be learned away from practice. 3 Discuss the role of reflection and critical incident analysis to enhance the quality of learning from experience.	Chapter 6. Refer to literature-based accounts of how decision making is learned. Examine a pre-registration nursing curriculum to identify where decision-making development is explicit.
6	Summary	Conclude the learning unit with a review of a continuum of decision-making expertise and approaches to teaching the development of decision-making skill.	1 Decide on an area for further study and pre-reading for the next learning unit (Chapter 7). 2 Make notes in your reflective diary about how you anticipate the nurse's decision-making role will develop in the future.	

Learning unit summary
By the end of this learning unit students will have examined concepts of expertise, a continuum of decision-making expertise, the concept of intellectual capital and ways of developing decision-making skill.

	Suggested areas for further study
1	*Defining expertise – comparing theory with practice* Conduct a literature search that is limited to a specific domain of clinical practice, and examine descriptions/definitions of decision-making expertise. Compare your findings with theoretical accounts in nurse education journals to determine to what extent practice understandings are explained by theoretical accounts of expert nursing and expert decision making. Would your description allow you to recognise an expert in your clinical area?
2	*Intellectual capital* How might you quantify the intellectual capital in the ward in which you work? What effects on patient care decision making can be detected when there are staff vacancies/losses from the clinical team? How can the intellectual capital of the team be enhanced?
3	*Skills of decision making* Examine your own role/person specification in order to identify what it states, if anything, about the required level of decision-making skill. If there is any evidence of this, what assumptions exist about how decisions are made and the skills that you need in order to make them? If it contains nothing about decision making, what would you include if you were rewriting this specification, and how would it alter the way in which you are portrayed as a nurse?

Learning Unit 7 Nurses as decision makers: where next?

Lesson aims
1 Examine decision accountability.
2 Examine and apply a narrative model as a method of demonstrating nurses' clinical decision making.
3 Examine and discuss the electronic record and its value in demonstrating decisions.

Text reference – Chapter 7.

Learning outcomes – 1 to 7.

	Learning content	Staff contribution	Student exercises	Learning resources
1	Introduction.	Having examined a range of issues about decision making this final learning unit examines decision accountability and considers how this might be achieved.	1 Recap learning and feedback from previous learning unit. 2 Students give feedback on their findings from their further study.	
2	Decision accountability.	Examine the framework of professional guidance on record keeping and professional accountability. Explore what nurses are accountable for and to whom.	Through group discussion develop an account of the range of accountability that a nurse has in the clinical workplace.	
3	How do you demonstrate clinical decisions?	Discuss methods of demonstrating decision process and decision outcomes. Use the narrative model as an analytical tool to analyse the text of a nursing decision (as shown in Chapter 7).	Examine how decisions are demonstrated in examples of nursing records.	Chapter 7. Examples of anonymised nursing records.

| 4 | Will the electronic record enhance the demonstration of clinical decision making? | Examine the design of an electronic health record. Discuss the underlying model and how this renders nurses' roles visible or invisible.

To what extent does the clinical team have access to electronically based decision support? Are there any barriers to accessing electronic information? If so, what are these and how can they be overcome? | Evaluate how the format of an electronic patient record will influence what is demonstrated about nurses' decisions.

Discuss whether all registered staff in identified clinical areas have the skills to search for and retrieve particular database information (e.g. best practice guidelines). To what extent can electronic information substitute for clinical experience and offset deficits in the intellectual capital of the ward team? | Examples of electronic patient record design (if available). |
| 5 | Module conclusion. | Review the module. Gather student feedback using a module evaluation questionnaire.

Discuss the module assignment. | 1 Complete module feedback questionnaire.
2 Discuss assignment preparation. | |

Learning unit summary

By the end of this learning unit students will have examined decision accountability and considered how this can be demonstrated.

Assignment

The completion of the module includes the submission of an assignment. Two options are suggested, one involving analysis of literature and the other involving analysis of a practice-based decision.

Suggested assignment: a literature review

A literature study of decision making in a chosen area of nursing practice

Guidance: Students are to select a chosen area of clinical practice (e.g. respiratory nursing, stroke nursing, Accident and Emergency nursing) and explain the rationale for their choice. They are to identify the search strategy they used to generate the results and the selection criteria they used to determine which papers to include in their study. The examination of the results needs to be structured around a conceptual framework. Using this, the assignment should explain the scope of existing enquiry in this field, the terminology used to explain nurses' decision making, and ways in which theory is used to explain how nurses make decisions. Examination of the literature should include a critique of reported differences and similarities in decision-making practice. In addition, it should include the decision-making context and its boundaries (e.g. legal, professional and organisational) and how these are visible in the literature examined. The conclusion of the assignment needs to identify gaps in existing enquiry and implications for future study.
Weighting: 100%.
Word limit: 3,000 words.

Suggested format of assignment

1 Title.
2 Introduction.
3 Search strategy and summary of results.
4 A conceptual framework.
5 Discussion of the different domains of the conceptual framework, to include:
 • decision-making definitions
 • theoretical explanations of decision making in this area
 • explanations of nurses as decision makers in this area
 • decision-making context.
6 Conclusion – include a summary and identify gaps in the existing field of enquiry.
7 References.

Suggested assignment: analysis of a clinical decision

An analysis of a real-world clinical decision

Guidance: Students are to identify and record an anonymised patient care decision and produce a chronological transcript of this. The decision will then be analysed. This should include the use of a conceptual framework to explain and examine the decision type, process, context, outcome and participants, and should specifically include examination of the roles of nurses in the decision and their interactions with non-nurses while making the decision. The analysis should also include an examination of the scope of decision making and nurses' decision authority. In addition, the analysis must include consideration of the role of formal and informal records, the decision context and how it shaped the process and subsequent decision made. Discuss the decision maker(s) and how their experience and knowledge shaped the decision process and outcome. The discussion section of the assignment should include a brief reflection on learning through having undertaken the analysis, and should identify how this will inform their approach to clinical decision-making practice.
Weighting: 100%.
Word limit: 3,000 words, excluding transcript.

Suggested format of assignment

1 Title.
2 Introduction.
3 Identification of the decision chosen.
4 A conceptual framework – this needs to include the decision participants, decision process, decision outcome and decision context. Explain how the framework will be used to examine the chosen decision example.
5 Analysis of the decision, to include:
   • decision process
   • formal and informal records
   • decision participants
   • decision outcome
   • decision context.
6 Discussion – include a reflection on learning drawn from the analysis and implications for clinical practice.
7 Conclusion.
8 References.
9 Appendix – transcript of the chosen decision.

Index